THE BEGINNER'S GUIDE
TO CRYSTAL HEALING

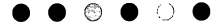

● ● ◉ ● ◯ ●

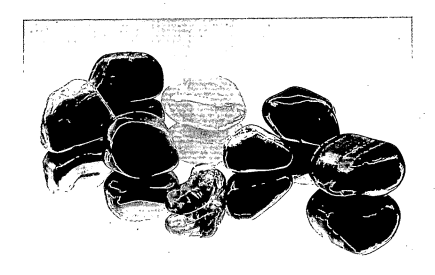

Shirley O'Donoghue

Healing Arts Press
Rochester, Vermont

Healing Arts Press
One Park Street
Rochester, Vermont 05767
www.HealingArtsPress.com

Healing Arts Press is a division of Inner Traditions International

Note to the reader: *This book is intended as an informational guide. The remedies, approaches, and techniques described herein are meant to supplement, and not to be a substitute for, professional medical care or treatment. They should not be used to treat a serious ailment without prior consultation with a qualified health care professional.*

Cataloging-in-Publication Data for this title is available from the Library of Congress

ISBN 978-1-64411-675-3 (print)
ISBN 978-1-64411-676-0 (ebook)

Printed and bound by Kultur Sanat Printing House, Turkey

10 9 8 7 6 5 4 3 2 1

Illustrations Phil O'Donoghue
Text design and layout Medlar Publishing Solutions Pvt. Ltd., India

To send correspondence to the author of this book, mail a first-class letter to the author c/o Inner Traditions • Bear & Company, One Park Street, Rochester, VT 05767, and we will forward the communication, or contact the author directly at **shirley@lucisgroup.com**

CONTENTS

PREFACE

This is a comprehensive guide to working with crystals. It is a useful resource for crystal therapists as well as practitioners of other therapies who would like to have a deeper understanding of crystals, so they can incorporate them into other treatments. It also offers a good foundation for non-practitioners who simply want to learn how they can use crystals to promote their own self-healing and personal and spiritual development, and will enable you to use and connect with crystals with confidence.

Interest in crystal therapy has grown considerably over the last few years and numerous books have been printed on the subject. With crystal therapy it is important to first understand that as everyone is different, individual responses to different crystals will vary from person to person, so learning to attune to crystals is key if you wish to work with crystals in a focused and effective manner.

I truly hope that this book will give you the confidence and techniques to get the most out of your crystals.

Best wishes,

Shirley O'Donoghue
Principal of Lucis College

ACKNOWLEDGMENTS

I would like to thank Sheila Corner and Wendy Hardiman-Evans for wading through the manuscript, giving advice on jewelry-making, and providing their insights into this book from a beginner's perspective. I'm glad that reading it has encouraged both Sheila and Wendy to expand their knowledge and delve into this amazing subject a little more.

Thank you to my astrologer friend—Pauline Gerosa (www.paulinegerosaastrology. com)—for her wise guidance on all things astrological.

Many thanks also to Vanessa Sutehall, who has given support and encouragement as well as feedback from an experienced crystal therapist's perspective. I'm really happy she found it inspired her too.

Thanks to all the hundreds of students I have had over the years, who have taught me just as much as I have taught them.

And, finally, thanks to my long-suffering husband Phil, who has helped with the illustrations and been on this book's journey with me every step of the way.

● ● ◌ ● ◌ ●

CHAPTER 1

CRYSTAL-THERAPY BASICS

THE HISTORY OF CRYSTAL THERAPY AND ATLANTIS

The use of crystals for healing purposes can be traced back in history to many ancient civilizations.

Egyptians used to bury their dead with quartz crystals placed on the brow (possibly on the brow chakra), and they wore amulets carved or decorated with stones such as lapis lazuli, carnelian, and turquoise. They also used crystals as cosmetics, grinding stones

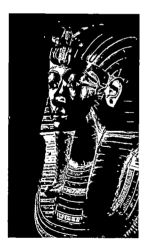

Tutankhamun's mask is decorated with crystals including lapis lazuli, quartz, obsidian, carnelian, and turquoise

such as galena into powders that they used as eye shadow—not a healthy cosmetic, as galena contains lead!

In China, jade was historically used to make death masks, musical instruments, and jewelry, and jade is still highly valued

there today. It was also considered to have healing properties and thought to be able to cure kidney stones. Chinese medicine incorporated crystals in the needles used in acupuncture.

The ancient Greeks believed that clear quartz remained solid because, buried deep in the earth, it had been frozen for so long that it would never melt. Many crystals' names come from the Greek. They made drinking cups and amulets out of amethyst—the Greek word *amethystos* means "not drunken."

The ancient Ayurvedic system of healing, which originated in India over two thousand years ago, is linked with the Hindu Veda scriptures, which document specific crystals

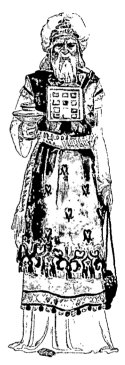

Carnelian breastplate, as mentioned in the book of Exodus

for their healing capabilities. Jasper was recommended to be used on the base chakra, much as some modern-day crystal therapists would use specific stones as a chakra set (more on this later).

The Mayans are reputed to have created thirteen crystal skulls, which were repositories of knowledge. Film culture today has referenced these skulls in *Indiana Jones and the Kingdom of the Crystal Skull*. The inspiration for the film was the discovery by the explorer F. A. Mitchell Hedges and his daughter Anna of the now-famous Mitchell Hedges Crystal Skull, which they found while excavating ancient Mayan ruins. There is a crystal skull that currently resides in the British Museum, two located in Paris, and another at the Smithsonian, all of which are surrounded by various myths and legends.

The list of cultures and civilizations continues with well-documented examples of the attributed healing/spiritual connection with crystals, right up to the current time. Even today, crystals are symbols of power and prestige—from bishops wearing amethyst rings to the diamonds studded into the Crown Jewels of the British monarchy. Religions around the world have acknowledged crystals, including carnelian breastplates mentioned in the Bible's book of Exodus for protection, the Koran describing the fourth heaven as made of garnet, Hindu writings describing the Kalpa Tree being made entirely of precious crystals, and Buddhist texts mentioning a throne made of diamond sited next to the Tree of Knowledge.

Stones were used alongside herbal medicine until the Renaissance, but as the scientific revolution evolved crystals as therapeutic/spiritual tools fell out of favor.

In the early 1980s, there was what could be called the dawning of the New Age, with authors such as Katrina Raphaell and Melody pioneering a combination

INTERESTING INFORMATION

Atlantis

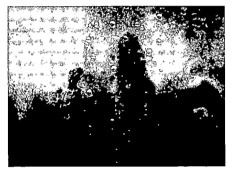

Atlantis

No one really knows if Atlantis is a myth or a real civilization that sank beneath the ocean (purportedly a punishment from the gods for its immorality). However, the name "Atlantean" was given by the Greeks to the Phoenician colonies along the Barbary Coast of North Africa. The first recorded acknowledgement of Atlantis was in unfinished writings of the ancient Greek philosopher Plato.

Some people who work with crystals believe that Atlantis holds the origins of crystal therapy. Modern-day psychics such as Edgar Cayce (1877–1945) have reinvigorated interest in the Atlantean mythology.

of old traditions with new ideas and techniques, once again raising awareness of crystal therapy.

Crystal therapy today, although far from being mainstream, continues to flourish, with a growing interest from both complementary therapists and beauty therapists. I hope that the coming years will see it become more accepted into mainstream therapy, as has happened with reiki and reflexology.

Crystals are a holistic treatment—their main strength lies in affecting the subtle energy that circulates throughout the energy systems. According to different ancient healing systems, this subtle energy consists of meridians, chakras, the aura, etc. The energy is sometimes known as prana, chi, or life- force energy, and if it becomes out of balance, holistic therapists accept that the effects can sometimes filter through and affect the physical body. This is the true core of holistic healing—affecting the mind, body, and soul—and is the basis of many of the ancient healing systems, such as Ayurveda and Chinese medicine, which are still practiced today.

CONTRAINDICATIONS FOR CRYSTAL THERAPY

There are some instances where crystal therapy treatments should be undertaken with caution.

When treating someone with epilepsy, care should be taken not to place crystals around the head. This is due to the electromagnetic charge that many crystals emit.

If you are treating someone with a mental illness such as psychosis or paranoia, the effects of a crystal treatment, although profoundly relaxing, can cause "spiritual" experiences such as a deep meditative state, visions, or other sensations. If patients are concerned or frightened by this potential, you should work very carefully with them.

With people who are using or have used mind-altering medications or drugs (even if this was some time ago), this may have opened neural pathways in the brain or led to a more open and receptive pineal gland, which means they are more likely to have a spiritual experience during crystal treatment. If they are stable, and if you feel confident you can rationalize and explain some of these responses, then this should not be a contraindication.

You should ask clients whether they have a pacemaker (and, if so, where exactly it is located) before giving treatment so that you can avoid that area. The minimal piezoelectrical charge of crystals could disrupt the pacemaker.

Some crystal therapists consider that a treatment should not be performed on a woman in the first trimester of her pregnancy. I personally feel that if things are progressing normally, and if the client understands about vibrational healing, there shouldn't really be a problem.

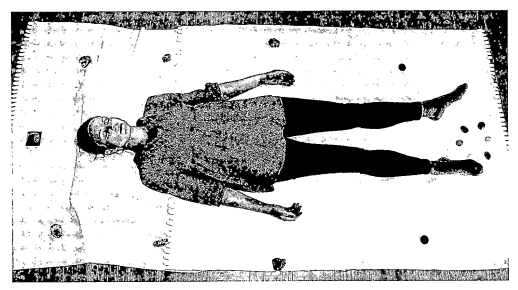

Patient surrounded by crystal grid

WHAT IS CRYSTAL HEALING?

• • • • • • • □ □ ○ • • • • ◡ ◻ . • • •

Crystal therapy, in the modern-day sense, is much more than wearing ornate jewelry, incorporating crystals into artefacts of power, or grinding them into powders to be ingested. Today, true crystal therapy is practiced as the placing of crystals on or around the body. Where the crystals are placed will determine whether they will work on the aura that surrounds the body,

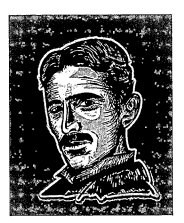

Nikola Tesla

on specific chakras, or even on acupressure or meridian points. I believe that crystals act as batteries that can realign, rebalance, energize, or unblock the invisible life-force energy that permeates the physical body via the subtle energy system. Many people, whether self-taught or professionally trained, begin to work with crystals by balancing chakras. This technique is explained in chapter 5.

So, how do they work? The honest answer is that no one really knows, although I believe that we are very near to quantum physics explaining the answer. Nikola Tesla was a Croatian inventor who for a short time worked with Thomas Edison in the United States. His inventions were ahead of their time, and whilst he was alive he never really got recognition for his work. Tesla was working in the early 1900s with the theory that everything has a frequency and vibration, and this is accepted by quantum physics today.

Modern science acknowledges that crystals have a form of energy that can alter vibrational resonances of other forms of energy (e.g., in our physical body). Put more simply, some exponents of crystal therapy say that the constant unwavering frequency (piezoelectricity) of a crystal interacts with the chaotic vibration given off by the human body (which is affected by so many things, such as our diet and our emotional and mental state). This constant, unchanging frequency brings order to an energy system that is often out of balance, and some would say chaotic.

INTERESTING CRYSTAL FACTS

- In the very rare rose quartz points, the inside of the crystal is made up of thousands of tiny points that have overgrown one another. This formation is known as a "massive."
- Pyrite is a source of sulfur.
- Elestial quartz is sometimes known as "cathedral quartz."
- The color of topaz can be changed by heat. Pure topaz is colorless, like clear quartz, but when it is irradiated (exposed to radiation) and heated it can turn different colors, such as blue and yellow.
- Jasper is a type of chalcedony (which is a type of quartz) that contains up to 20% impurities, which help to determine its color, streak, and appearance.
- Carnelian is a variety of chalcedony.
- Garnet is used as a grinding/polishing agent as well as in jewelry.
- Hematite can become tarnished, shatters easily, and can irritate the skin.
- Malachite is very toxic when it is ground; never breathe in malachite dust.
- Sugilite is a purple stone that was discovered in 1944 by and is named after Japanese petrologist Ken-ichi Sugi, and is also known as luvulite.
- Obsidian occurs as crusts on lava flows. In the Stone Age, obsidian was a much-valued raw material for utensils and weapons owing to its sharp-edged fracture and hardness.
- Fluorite can fade when left in sunlight. It is used in toothpaste to help harden tooth enamel.
- Citrine has the same chemical constituents as amethyst—citrine occurs when the mix of mineral constituents has been subjected to extreme heat, either naturally or intentionally in the process to produce citrine. Ametrine is a combination of amethyst and citrine, and has brown/orange/yellow citrine inclusions within the purple amethyst.
- Lapis lazuli contains lazurite, pyrite, white calcite, and sodalite.
- Clear quartz is a raw material used in making glass and in the ceramic industry. In technological products it serves as a regulator (its vibration can be used to create an electrical signal with a precise frequency) and is used in radios, transmitters, and clocks, among other things.

Whether this will prove to be a satisfactory answer to how crystals work, only time will tell. So many cultures have, over the years, embraced crystals for their energies without scientific proof. I would argue that the concept of crystal therapy would not have lasted this long if they truly were inanimate objects.

Although nowadays the most common ways of using crystals are to carry them around in your pocket or wear them as an item of jewelry, this book will, I hope, open you to all sorts of other possibilities, as well as give you the confidence to work with crystal energy on deeper and deeper levels.

QUESTIONS ON CHAPTER 1

1. List three civilizations that identified and used crystals to promote power and authority or for their healing qualities.
2. Explain the myth of Atlantis and why it is relevant to crystal therapy.
3. Explain what a contraindication is and give three contraindications for crystal therapy.
4. Explain what crystal therapy is.

● ● ○ ● ◡ ●

CHAPTER 2

SELECTING AND TAKING CARE
OF YOUR CRYSTALS

HOW TO CHOOSE THE CORRECT CRYSTALS FOR YOU

Although it is commonly accepted that we choose the crystals that we need to work with, perhaps it is worth considering the possibility that the reality is the reverse of this: that in fact the crystal chooses us in order to gain the opportunity to work with the energy, healing, and spiritual-developmental requirements, for example, that we present.

Connecting with crystals can sometimes be a profoundly spiritual experience, and at other times very casual. We can feel an instant and profound energetic link, or simply be drawn to the color of the crystal. Either way, some healers feel that this connection is initiated by the crystalline intelligence rather than the reverse.

Buying a crystal is usually a very personal experience, and you should never be guided into buying a crystal purely because outside information tells you that it is appropriate for you. Equally, don't be deterred from getting a crystal that you are drawn to simply because the information that you get from a book or another person does not seem to "fit" what you are looking for.

Crystals are a bit like radio transmitters that transmit different stations—purely classical, pop, or jazz music, say, or talk stations where no music is played at all—on different frequencies. We are like the radio tuner that can access the different frequency waves. Therefore, people have differing perceptions of what specific energetic roles crystals can fulfil, and that is why it is so important for us as healers, firstly, to develop our intuition for ourselves, but, secondly, to expand our awareness in order to be able to "tune in" on behalf of our clients and assess their energetic requirements.

This is also the reason that crystal therapy is so difficult to communicate to the uninitiated, who might pick up several books or visit websites on crystals and find contradictory information in them.

As people become more aware of and interested in crystals, many suddenly realize that they have quickly amassed a collection of crystals and gems of differing shapes, sizes, and colors without having really gained an understanding of why those crystals have come to them in the first place, or even the types of crystals or their names.

What to consider when deciding to buy a crystal

Always pay attention to your first instincts and reactions, whether positive or negative. At this point, logic hasn't had time to step in, and the instinctive, intuitive part of you has an opportunity to communicate with you.

Balance the rational with the magical—if you are clearly not able to afford a crystal at a particular time, try sending a thought out to the universe to ask for the necessary financial energy for you to have the crystal, if it is appropriate for your highest good. Set a date, and return to the shop to see if the crystal is still waiting for you.

Take note of the crystals that you dislike as well as the ones that you are drawn to—this can provide information for you to work with.

A good shop will be able to give you information on any special storage or handling requirements of the crystals you buy. For example, amethyst should never be placed in direct sunlight as it will turn a brownish purple.

Crystals vary in their hardness. Some, therefore, are more delicate than others and easier to damage. Always ensure that you know the names of the crystals you are buying so that you can find out any special storage or other requirements that they have.

HOW TO DOWSE AND WHY

Many people who work on the subtle energy system learn the art of dowsing with a pendulum in order to monitor the patient's energy flow prior to a treatment, and to check the changes that have occurred during or after a treatment—in the dowsing fraternity this is known as "dowsing for health."

Dowsing is primarily associated with finding water sources, but it can also be used to find lost objects, to identify the best mineral supplements, or to identify environmental stressors, such as electromagnetic or geopathic stressors. Experienced dowsers often use specific instruments for these different activities, such as rods, but the traditional dowsing tool is the "Y"-shaped hazel branch. You can even make a set of rods from old wire coat hangers!

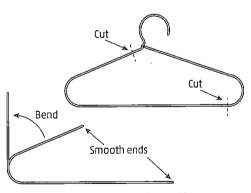

How to make a dowsing rod from a wire coat hanger

However, for our purposes, pendulums are the easiest tool to work with. These come in all shapes, sizes, and materials, so it is important to find one that works best for you.

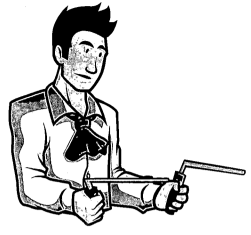

Using dowsing rods

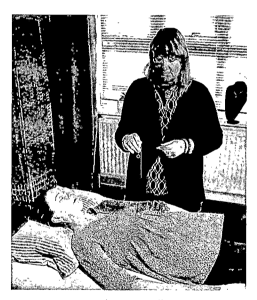

Dowsing over a client

Dowsing is something that anyone can learn to do. When you first begin it is important to try to keep yourself in a state of relaxed alertness—try not to feel under pressure to get the pendulum to move, and ensure that you are as comfortable as possible.

You now need to find out what the movement means for you. Everyone has a

different response from a pendulum, and so you need to discover what movements indicate *yes, no,* and *maybe* or *neutral*. Remember, it is important to simply accept what works for you.

Hold the pendulum so that your fingers are about 3–3½ inches (7.5–9 cm) from the weighted end. If there is any excess chain or string, ensure that it is held away from the weighted end so that it doesn't restrict the pendulum's movement.

Take a couple of deep breaths to relax, and ensure that you are centered and grounded. Don't try to dowse if you feel agitated or negative.

Mentally or aloud, ask the pendulum to show you your *yes* movement—wait for a few moments and you may be aware that the pendulum is shaking, or it may even start to move straight away.

Once it has moved, allow a little time for it to settle—it is not uncommon for it to start off slowly and build up speed. If you find that there is no movement, try holding the pendulum above the outstretched palm of your other hand (palm facing upwards), as this can sometimes help to "jump-start" it.

Once you have your *yes* response, stop the pendulum by holding it to still its movement, and repeat the exercise, this time asking for your *no* and then your *neutral* response.

The next step is simply to practice—you can ask questions that you know the answer to,

Maybe

Yes

No

Dowsing chart. There is a larger version of this chart in appendix 6 that you could photocopy.

and then move on to questions that you can check after you have received the answer from your pendulum. Done consistently, this will improve your ability to dowse and add to your confidence in it.

IMPORTANT NOTE: If you find you cannot dowse, this will not stop you from working with crystals and developing your sensitivity. But do persevere with this technique if you can.

INTERESTING INFORMATION

Did you know that there is an organization that promotes dowsing in the US? It is called the American Society of Dowsers and was founded in 1961. It aims to disseminate knowledge of dowsing, development of its skills, and recognition for its achievements. There is a similar organization in the UK, called the British Society of Dowsers, which has been in operation since 1933. It promotes the study and understanding of dowsing for health and well-being, water divining, archaeology, earth energies (ley lines, water lines), and so on.

CLEANSING CRYSTALS

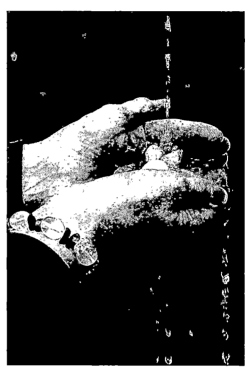

Washing crystals

It is extremely important that crystals are cleansed on a regular basis, for many reasons. When you first obtain a crystal you have no idea of who has handled it or how they were feeling at the time, or any trauma experienced by the crystal through the mining process (some crystals find their way into the light of day through massive explosions or are "cleaned" in acid, for example).

A crystal works by absorbing energy, whether it is negative or positive, and thereby rebalancing the energy field of the person handling it. So, it is possible to obtain a crystal that carries stagnant energy. As a responsible healer you will recognize this intuitively and be enabled to take steps to clear and attune the crystal back to its appropriate frequency. In the same way, if you were having a beauty treatment you would expect that the therapist would sterilize any equipment that had been used between clients to avoid the chance of cross-contamination. A crystal may be imbued with positive energy, but I feel it important that when using a crystal in a treatment it should be as clear as possible of outside influences so that it can work effectively with the individual energy of the person receiving the treatment.

Healers develop a feel for when a crystal needs to be cleansed. The crystal may seem a little dull and lifeless, or you may just feel instinctively that it should be cleansed. You can try using a pendulum to show you whether a cleansing procedure is required, or it may simply be that you carry out a cleansing routine of your own each time you select a crystal as well as when you have finished working with it.

The frequency of cleansing required seems to vary from healer to healer and crystal to crystal. Obviously, crystals that are working hard need to be cleansed more frequently, but remember that if a crystal is sitting in a room where the atmosphere is continually negative it will still be absorbing this energy even though you are not consciously handling it.

Should you find that a crystal does not respond to cleansing it may be because it needs to recuperate, or, more rarely, has been misused in the past. It is best in these cases to leave the crystal to rest and continue to monitor it from time to time. Another possible reason is that it has finished its work with you and wishes to move on. This usually results in the healer being inspired to pass the crystal on to someone else, which is unfortunately an expensive practice that most healers encounter with varying degrees of resistance, although that resistance is usually futile!

When you initially cleanse a crystal you have just obtained, you can use this opportunity to ritualize the process in order to become acquainted more closely with the crystal and to gain a better understanding of what it has connected with you to achieve. After this first time, the process of cleansing does not need to be so intense.

Here are some ideas for cleansing crystals—again, go with what feels right and appropriate for you. If you are empowered to make up your own ways of cleansing, then please follow them.

Holding crystals under running water: this can be tap water, local spring water, sea waves, etc. It is important to check that the crystals are suitable to be placed in water. Some, such as gypsum, can become fragile in water, and halite is a salt crystal that will dissolve if left in water.

Visualization: this is a way of helping your mind focus on only one thing. Make up whatever seems appropriate. It might be a visualization of white light flooding through the crystal, clearing out any stagnant energy, for example. If you are confident with visualization you can cleanse an entire collection of crystals, and do not even have to be present in the room when you are carrying out the visualization.

Using sound, chanting, Tibetan bowls, etc.: you can either hold the crystal or place it in front of you.

Placing in sunlight, moonlight, rain, etc.: you can simply leave crystals out in the elements and collect them later. Allow your intuition to tell you when the process has finished.

Soaking in a solution of salt and water or gem essence.

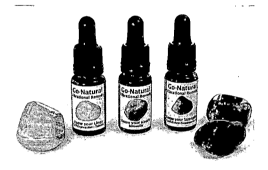

Gem-essences

Burying crystals in the ground: the length of time they are kept underground is down to your intuitive feelings. Personally, I have never felt drawn to use this method, but I know crystal therapists who do.

Burying crystals in or passing them through salt: do take care when using this process as salt is also a crystal and may scratch softer crystals—see the section on the Mohs scale under Crystal Attunement Sheets in chapter 3 for more information.

The hardness level of a crystal determines whether it can damage or be damaged by other crystals. Crystals that are graded as softer will be damaged by crystals that are graded harder on the Mohs scale. You should avoid placing crystals alongside one another in a bag, for example, where they can rub against each other, causing chipping or scratching.

INTERESTING INFORMATION

Common Natural Crystal Formations and How Their Shape Influences the Crystal's Energy

1. Acicular—needle-like crystals said to remove negative energy.

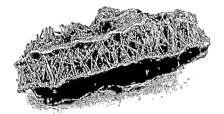

Acicular formation

2. Crystal termination or point—if the crystal's base is placed against the body it will draw off energy, if reversed it will direct energy towards the body, so this shape is good for unblocking and energizing chakras, meridians, etc.

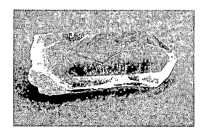

Quartz point

3. Pyramid—creates a grounding energy that also focuses upward. This shape also creates a large energy field around it, which can be protective and supportive.

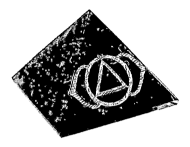

Pyramid

4. Cubic—grounds and consolidates energy.

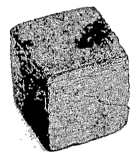

Cubic formation

5. Cluster—radiates energy in all directions; a good crystal shape to hold the energy in a room.

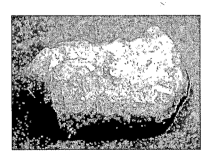

Cluster formation

6. Geode—amplifies while generating energy.

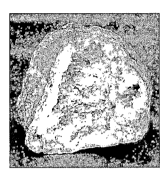

Geode

7. Double terminated—generates energy in two directions, accelerating connections with others or between spirit realms and physical realms.

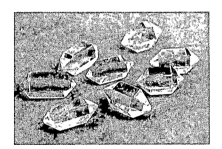

Double-terminated crystals

8. Elestial—sometimes known as cathedral quartz, this shape is said to open doorways to change, and to be excellent for connection to spiritual realms, angels, and the akashic (past-life) records.

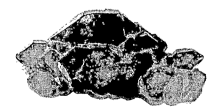

Elestial formation

These formations are less common, and could be considered abnormalities of growth:

1. Tabby or tabular crystal—excellent crystals to generate healing and information connected to the earth.

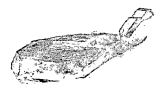

Tabby quartz

2. Bridge crystal—as the name suggests, it creates a bridge between two worlds in any areas of our lives where we need a bridge—e.g., inner/outer world, physical/spiritual, etc.

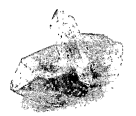

Bridge crystal

3. Candle quartz—considered to be an excellent crystal for lightworkers who are helping to change the energy of the planet. Heals ancestral lines and karmic inheritance.

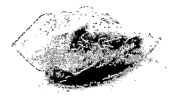

Candle quartz

4. Scepter quartz crystal—directs energy and also an ideal crystal to use in ceremonies and rituals as it helps to focus group energy. Is also said to empower healing generally.

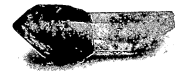

Scepter quartz

5. Laser crystal—slender and delicate to look at, the laser configuration is said to be a high vibrational crystal, which can be used as a powerful healing tool.

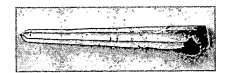

Laser crystal

Tuning into Different Shapes

If you want to attune to the energy of different shapes and forms of crystals, gather together either crystals that are different types but have the same shape as one another, or the same type of crystal but in a variety of different shapes. Just hold them one at a time in your hand for a few moments with your eyes closed, and simply "sit" with the energy. Record your responses to each crystal—you will be surprised how different they feel.

QUESTIONS ON CHAPTER 2

1. Describe three ways of choosing crystals for healing. Give the advantages and disadvantages of each method you choose.
2. Explain what dowsing is and how you can use it to select crystals.
3. Give two theories as to why crystals need cleansing.
4. Describe four methods of cleansing crystals, giving the advantages and disadvantages of each. What is your favorite method of cleansing crystals, and why?

● ● ○ ● ⟩ ●

CHAPTER 3

GETTING TO KNOW YOUR CRYSTALS

I and many other crystal users are convinced that crystals do absorb our thoughts and feelings, although I personally don't often program a crystal to do what I want.
I prefer to connect with the crystal and to gain an understanding of how it is happy to connect with me. For those who feel that their intuitive ability is not quite enough, it is possible to use a pendulum or simply to ask. This, I feel, is working from a basis of mutual respect and cooperation. Obviously, when moderating the activity of a crystal there is a karmic aspect to that act. In making a crystal "do" what you want it to, it could be argued that you may take away the free will of the crystal. Therefore, it is important to develop your ability to attune to crystals so that working with them becomes a partnership between you and the crystals.

Before starting the following procedures, cleanse the crystal.

DEDICATING A CRYSTAL
● ● ● ● ● ● ● ○ ○ ○ ● ● ● ● ⟩ ⟩ ⟩ ● ● ● ●

Whenever you work with a crystal for the first time, it is important to affirm that you wish the crystal to work from a position of the highest good.

I usually say something along the lines of: "May this crystal work for the good of all and the harm of none, and may it work for the highest and purist good." What we are doing when we dedicate a crystal is asking that it is sanctified and blessed to work in the name of love and light.

ATTUNING TO A CRYSTAL
● ● ● ● ● ● ● ○ ○ ● ● ● ● ○ ⟩ ● ● ● ●

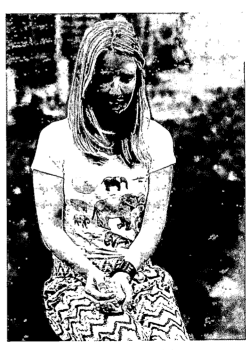

Attuning to a crystal

Take time to follow this procedure when you first start working with crystals. Soon you will find that the process becomes quicker and you will be able to connect with a crystal after a few seconds.

Sit quietly, holding the crystal in your "receiving hand" (this is usually the left, and the right hand is usually considered to be the "giving hand," but follow your own intuition). Try to connect with the crystal in any way that is appropriate, using visualization, sensing the energy, or simply asking the crystal to "tell" you how it wishes to work with you. You may find that the response comes in the form of inner knowing, words that drop into your mind without conscious thought, heightened emotion, or pictures in your mind. When the process is complete, honor and acknowledge the help that you have received, both from the crystal kingdom and from your guides.

As you develop your sensitivity to crystals you will become more confident and able to accept, more confidently, the forms in which these supposedly inanimate objects can communicate with us.

Attuning your crystals will allow you to work more effectively. Below is a list of common crystals that are easy and affordable to obtain. They are stones that are very popular with crystal therapists, but feel free to use whichever crystals you have available.

See appendix 1 (Crystal Glossary) for pictures of each crystal listed below:

Amber	Pyrite
Amethyst	Blue quartz
Aventurine	Clear quartz
Carnelian	Rose quartz
Citrine	Smoky quartz
Hematite	Snowy quartz
Red jasper	Sodalite
Lapis lazuli	Tiger's eye
Malachite	Black tourmaline
Moonstone	Turquoise
Snowflake obsidian	

When you attune to a crystal, it is helpful to complete a crystal attunement sheet.

CRYSTAL ATTUNEMENT SHEETS

Attunement sheets are guidelines to support you as you meditate and connect with your crystals. You will gain a lot of insight by researching for yourself information about the crystals and their geological correspondences, chemical composition, countries they are mined in, colors, crystal system, and so on, as well as recording other people's perspectives of crystal uses alongside a good selection of esoteric meanings for crystals—all of this information can be found in books and on the internet. This will create a foundation on which you can build a stronger, closer connection to your crystals to enhance however you choose to work with them.

Listed below are some explanatory notes that should help you complete the attunement sheets. You will be able to find the crystallography information in any good

---

CRYSTAL ATTUNEMENT SHEET

Your interpretation of the significance and uses of this crystal – *give at least three:*

Crystal Name:	**Family Group Name:**
Crystal System:	**Chemical Composition:**
Countries of Origin:	**Hardness:**
Crystal Formation:	
Colors:	

Other Significant Information – Special care, poisonous, contra-indications:

Meanings – from at least three different sources: please continue overleaf

---

geology book from the library or a good bookstore. However, nowadays it is easier to get the appropriate information by simply searching on the internet.

Family group name

Some crystals can be grouped together into families—for example, rose quartz, amethyst, clear quartz, and citrine are all members of the quartz family. This is what is known as the family group name. Other crystals, such as celestite and sugilite, are not part of a family and are referred to by their initial name only.

Crystal system

The "crystal system" refers to the crystal lattice structure—the three-dimensional way in which the atoms of the crystal are arranged. There are seven systems—

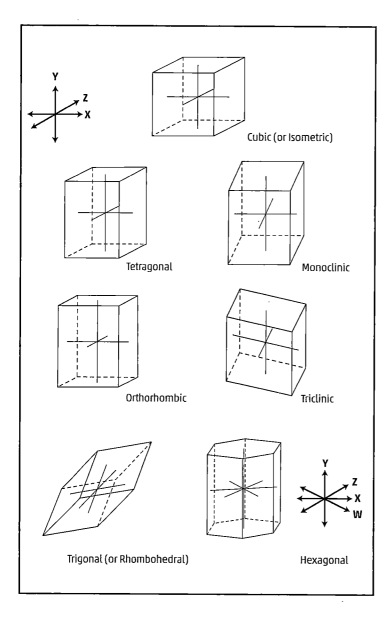

The seven crystal systems. Cubic: All axes are at right angles to one another, and are of equal length. Tetragonal: All axes are at right angles to one another but only two of the three axes are equal in length. Orthorhombic: All axes are at right angles to one another and are unequal in length. Monoclinic: Only two axes are at right angles to each other and all three axes are unequal in length. Triclinic: All axes are unequal in length and not at right angles to one another. Trigonal: Crystal faces all have the same size and shape and axes are of equal length but none of the axes are at right angles to one another. Hexagonal: Of the four axes only three are of equal length. The fourth axis, "Y," is at 90° to the other three.

tetragonal, trigonal, hexagonal, cubic, monoclinic, orthorhombic, and triclinic.

Note that some stones will not be part of a crystal system and may be known as "rocks" or termed "amorphous."

Chemical composition

This refers to the different constituents of a crystal. This may be of interest particularly if you are considering preparing gem essences, or elixirs (see box), looking at the ways that crystals can interact with the human energy system. You do not need to provide the exact chemical formula—listing the ingredients is enough.

Hardness

Frederick Mohs created the Mohs scale, which classifies the hardness of different crystals. It starts at 1, which is the softest and includes crystals such as talc, and goes up to 10, which includes diamonds. A good point of reference is that a fingernail is classified as 4, which means that your fingernails can scratch any crystal classified as 4 or below. Therefore, it is important to store your crystals separately, preferably in boxes with compartments so that they don't rub against one another and get scratched or damaged. You can also label them, and this will also gradually help you to be able to identify the most suitable cleansing rituals.

GEM ELIXIRS

Making a gem elixir is a simple and effective way of using crystal energy. Scientists are beginning to find that water can hold and store energetic vibrations from flowers, the environment, color, crystals, etc. The flower essences in the world-famous Bach range are created by leaving flowers in spring water in sunlight for several hours and then preserving that water with brandy. Similarly, you can place a crystal in water and after a period the water will absorb some of the qualities of the crystal into itself—thus you can create a rose quartz essence in

this way, for example. You can dowse to check when the water has absorbed the energy from the crystal and the process is complete. See chapter 7 for more information.

IMPORTANT NOTE: If you would like to work with crystals in this way it is vital that you ensure that the crystals you are using are not toxic—like arsenic or cinnabar—and that they are not damaged by being immersed in water. There is a section on toxic crystals in chapter 7, but do double-check with your retailer.

Mohs Hardness Scale		
Mineral Name	Scale Number	Scratch Test
Talc	1	Can be scraped with fingernail
Gypsum	2	Can be scratched with fingernail
Calcite	3	Can be scratched with copper coin
Fluorite	4	Can be scratched easily with knife
Apatite	5	Can be scratched with knife
Orthoclase	6	Can be scratched with steel file
Quartz	7	Scratches window glass
Topaz	8	Scratches quartz
Corundum	9	Scratches topaz
Diamond	10	Scratches corundum

The Mohs hardness scale

INTERESTING INFORMATION

Crystal Systems and Their Correspondences

When choosing a crystal, you might want to consider the impact that its crystal system has on its energy. Here's an overview of how your crystal is affected by its internal structure:

The **trigonal system** relates best to the base chakra. This system is excellent for aligning the subtle bodies and bringing clarity. These crystals include amethyst, quartz, tourmaline.

The **cubic system** relates best to the sacral chakra, and this system helps to generate a grounding energy that helps to inspire on a mundane, lower level, so these crystals are good for supporting basic earthly needs and emotions. The crystals include pyrite, fluorite, diamond.

The **hexagonal system** is linked to the solar plexus, and these crystals are great for providing energy and vitality as well as supporting intuitive development. The crystals include aquamarine, beryl, emerald.

The **tetragonal system** works with the heart chakra. This system is a natural balancer of energy. These crystals are a bridge between heaven and earth. The crystals include apophyllite, rutile, wulfenite.

The **orthorhombic system** is connected to the throat chakra, and the orthorhombic system helps to magnify, support, and release by providing perspective and focus. These crystals include peridot, aragonite, topaz.

The **monoclinic system** is aligned to the brow chakra. This system is excellent as a support for meditation and clearing the brow chakra from mental chatter so that you can connect more easily to higher spiritual energies. These crystals include azurite, jade, malachite.

The **triclinic system** is linked to the crown chakra, and this system generates harmony and spiritual awareness. These crystals include labradorite, sunstone, rhodonite.

Crystal formation

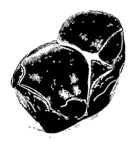

Botroidal formation

· This relates to the ways that crystals are formed—in other words, the ways that they grow—and some geological books refer to this as "crystal habits." For example, rose quartz is usually found as "massive" pieces of rock (crystal clusters have been found, but they are very rare and usually extremely small). Clear quartz is mainly found in groups (or clusters), single crystals (or terminations), or double-terminated prismatic crystals, although it is also sometimes found in chunks, or "massive" formations.

Colors

Some crystals have a single color, but others come in a range of different colors. For example, tourmaline comes in black, green, pink, yellow, or blue, or with a mixture of colors such as in watermelon tourmaline.

Other significant information

In this section you should include anything that you feel may be of interest. For example, if a crystal is poisonous or very soft you may wish to note this so that when making gem elixirs you do not make the essence by placing the crystal in water. (A gem elixir captures the energy of the crystal in water, which allows you to use the elixir in similar ways to the Bach flower remedies.)

This section can also be used to note identifying factors that you find of interest, or any special contraindications.

Traditional meanings

These relate to the information that you have resourced from other authors on the qualities that a crystal has, as well as historical beliefs relating to the crystal. Please note that you do not have to agree with other authors' interpretations, but you may see a correspondence with the information, such as an opposing perspective.

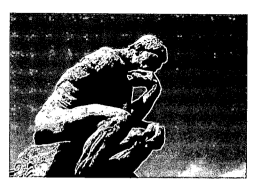

The Thinker

Your interpretation

This is arguably the most important section on an attunement sheet. This section is designed to allow you to develop your own perceptions of the qualities that certain crystals hold for you. It should be noted that what results from your attunement practices is individual to you, and you should do these attunements by meditating or working with the crystals—preferably both.

When you attune to a crystal, this allows your energy and the energy of the stone to vibrate in harmony. This process helps you to develop a bond with the crystal, whilst also understanding how it is affecting the energies of the room or client it is connecting with.

MEDITATING TO ATTUNE TO A CRYSTAL

Firstly, hold the crystal in your hand and really look at it. Observe the color, shape, inclusions, and so on. How does it reflect the light? What size is it? What other visible features does it have? Some people believe that your left hand is the best hand to receive energies and perceptions from the crystals—this may be related to the left side of the body being linked to the right side of the brain (the left brain is considered rational and analytical, and right side of the brain is thought to be intuitive and creative). Close your eyes and try to remember what the crystal looked like in your mind's eye. Now feel your stone and become aware of its temperature and shape—is it rough or smooth? Become aware of any thoughts that just seem to pop into your mind from nowhere, and try holding the stone on chakra points to see if you can feel the connection at any chakras. Pay attention to colors that appear in your third eye and any emotional sensations that well up—again, seemingly from nowhere.

Now, bringing your focus back into the room, write down any thoughts, feelings, or perceptions that have occurred while you have carried out this process. It is important not to judge these. Once you have completed this exercise, then either reference your findings with other crystal practitioners (you can do this by discussing it with like-minded friends who have carried out the same exercise), compare your findings to those found in any crystal books you have, or alternatively just Google your crystal's name on the internet and see what comes up—you will be astonished as you practice and master this process to find how similar your perceptions are to others'—coincidence or not?

Being in harmony with your stone makes it much easier for the two of you to work together. The more attuned you are to your stones, the better they will work for you, and the deeper your connection will be.

ENERGIZING AND CHARGING CRYSTALS

Energizing and charging crystals are similar procedures in that they provide additional

	Sunlight	Masculine, Fiery, Energising, Powerful
	Moonlight	Feminine, Dark, Secret, Intuitive, Calm
	Angelic	Compassion, Love, Ceremony, Guidance
	Starlight	Manifesting, Cosmic Awareness, Multidimensional
	Storm	Elemental, Transformational, Rebirth
	Earth	Groundedness, Womblike, Replenishing, Healing
	Water	Cleansing, Emotional Release
	Fire	Movement, Personal Power, Purification
	Air	Freedom, Spirit, Breath

Crystal charging qualities table

energy to the crystal. Energizing can be as simple as asking for the crystal to operate at the optimum level of its capacity, and it can be a technique used to help heal and clear a crystal that has been damaged or has had to work very hard. Charging is slightly different in that we can supply the crystal with a specific type of energy—for example, solar, lunar, storm, or angelic. (Many people believe that while we have guides who are here to lead and teach us lessons that we have been incarnated in this lifetime to learn, the role of the angelic hierarchy is to offer us love and support in times of difficulty. Energizing your crystal with angelic frequency will allow the crystal to generate this love and support in addition to the other qualities it holds.) The time that you need to spend energizing a crystal will vary enormously and you should go by your intuition, or you could dowse to ask whether the process has finished. You simply leave the crystal to soak up the energetic quality of the element you feel is appropriate, and go back to collect it when it has been charged.

It is also possible to charge your crystal with reiki energy (or any other form of healing energy) by simply holding the crystal and allowing the reiki to flow from your hands into the crystal. Hold the crystal until the energy from your hands slows or stops, and that will indicate that the crystal has absorbed as much of the reiki as it requires.

SELF-HEALING WITH CRYSTALS—ENERGY FLUSH

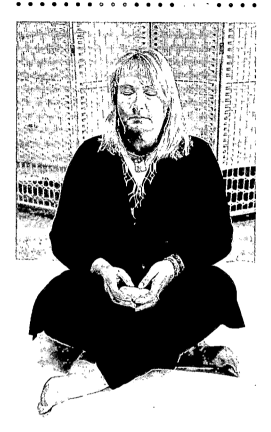

Self-healing

You will need: two quartz points.

Timing: around 10 minutes.

Technique: Hold one quartz point in your left hand, pointing up your arm, and hold the other point in your right hand, pointing away from your right arm. Sit or lie and try to focus on breathing in through the nose and out through the mouth. As you do this, visualize clear white energy flowing through the crystal point you are holding in your left hand, and see it moving up your arm, into the shoulder, and then flowing throughout your body. As the energy flows, become aware that it is clearing stagnant energy from your chakras and meridians within the subtle energy system, along with your aura. Allow the energy to flow throughout your physical and energy bodies, and as it continues its journey visualize it being guided into your right shoulder and flowing down your right arm, before being drawn away by the crystal point in your right hand.

When you have finished, put the crystals down and open your eyes. Bring yourself back to ordinary everyday awareness.

QUESTIONS ON CHAPTER 3

1. What is the difference between attuning to and dedicating a crystal?
2. Think about how you would energize and charge a crystal. Give examples of types of crystals you have charged with different energies, and describe how you feel the crystal's energy responded to this process.
3. Complete attunements to at least five crystals. Once you have attuned to each crystal, reference your findings against other descriptions of crystal properties—possible authors could include July Hall, Melody, etc., or you can Google crystal healing properties on the Web.

CHAPTER 4

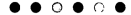

THE LINK BETWEEN COLOR AND CRYSTALS

COLOR THERAPY AND CRYSTALS

Each culture has its own understanding of the meanings of different colors. In the West, our instinct is that red is vibrant, symbolizing passion and danger, while green is healthy and represents new growth. Different cultures, however, attach very different meanings to colors, yet color is simply light of different wavelengths and frequencies. The visible spectrum consists of seven colors of the rainbow, and each color has its own wavelength and frequency. We are all surrounded by electromagnetic waves of energy of which color is just a small part.

For example, red excites the senses and is at one end of the spectrum (wavelength 700 nanometers), while blue is cooling and calming and is at the other end of the spectrum (400 nanometers). The energy relating to each of these spectrum colors resonates with the energy of one of the seven main chakras of the body.

Historical and archaeological evidence from varied and different civilizations shows that people have always been fascinated and intrigued by color; even today we are still exploring its effects on our surroundings and ourselves.

Those who believe that the mythical island of Atlantis existed believe that Atlanteans used color to treat and enhance themselves and their surroundings. For others who take a more grounded viewpoint, the use of color to treat ailments has been traced back to ancient Egypt. The ancient Egyptians were a people who worshipped the earth and the planets, and they used green on the floors of many of their temples. There is a link with the modern use of therapeutic color, as they created different rooms in specific colors for spiritual and healing purposes, harnessing the power of the sun, which they worshipped as a deity, to illuminate and energize the colors. They were also aware of the therapeutic uses that crystals and gems could be put to.

Although there are written lists dating as far back as 1550 BC giving color "cures," a great deal of this knowledge may have been lost with the advent of ancient Greek civilization, when color became regarded as a science. The practice of using color as a therapeutic tool, however, was handed down

INTERESTING INFORMATION

It was the ancient Greeks who first took a more scientific stance, with Plato and Pythagoras studying the effects of light, and Aristotle combining two colors to produce a third. He was reputed to have illustrated this using two pieces of glass, one yellow and the other blue. When these were overlaid, he produced green—an effect many young schoolchildren could testify to.

In Europe, Paracelsus brought the subject to prominence again in the Middle Ages.

As color healers are aware, white light is made up of all the colors of the spectrum (red, orange, yellow, green, blue, indigo, and violet)—quartz is considered to hold the qualities of all the colors, and works as a "white-light" crystal.

by a very few people. There are also records of the Chinese using color therapeutically nearly two thousand years ago.

Each color has a specific meaning, and the color wheel is made up of the primary colors—red, yellow, and blue—and the secondary colors—orange, green, and purple (these are called secondary colors because they are products of mixing two primary colors together). Your instinct may be to identify with the qualities of the colors listed below, to make a connection with the colors in terms of chakra correspondences, or a combination of both—whatever feels appropriate for you.

Note that green is complementary to red, orange is complementary to blue, and yellow is complementary to violet.

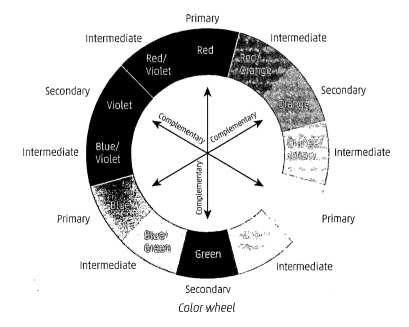

Color wheel

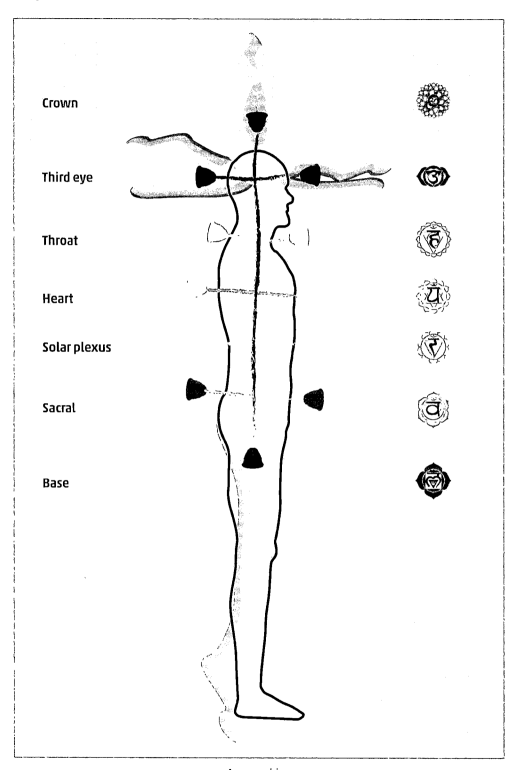

Crown

Third eye

Throat

Heart

Solar plexus

Sacral

Base

Aura machine

The human energy field, or aura, is composed of subtle energies that some people can perceive as color. People who can see these colors in our energy fields report that they can shift and change rapidly—affected by emotions, thoughts, or activity. They can also be affected by health changes. There is usually a dominant color contained within each energy field, which varies from person to person.

Although there is known to be bioelectrical activity within the body, which activates nerves and muscles but is not visible to the naked eye, science is starting to speculate that the body also has an electromagnetic field (or aura, as the ancients would call it) that responds to the electromagnetic energy given from tools such as crystals and color, albeit on a subtle vibration.

HOW LIGHT IS REFLECTED THROUGH CRYSTALS

When we look at a green crystal, although we see the color green the crystal is actually reflecting green away from itself, and in reality the green crystal is holding on to the other six colors of the spectrum to varying degrees.

COLOR CORRESPONDENCES

Each color has a different correspondence.

Commonly accepted color correspondences

Understanding more about color correspondences can help you to select a crystal effectively. It is important to note that there are no good or bad colors; however, each color presents with a negative and positive aspect. You will also see that while some crystals are a specific color, they will resonate with a few chakras rather than just one.

The following outlines some of the aspects of each color.

Red

Red is action-oriented and represents drive and energy. It can strengthen will power and promote courage, focus, and vitality. Use it for someone who is depressed and lacks vitality. However, it should not be used when the person is angry or stressed.

Other keywords: passion, life, blood, strength, happiness, love, hate, summer, fire, sexual desire, the Maiden, independence, courage, truthfulness, fever, the South, physical growth, ambition, aggression, assertiveness, achieving goals.

Red stones: garnet, ruby, red jasper, red aventurine, red phantom quartz.

Orange

Orange links to personal power and strengthens determination. It is seen as a lucky color and dissipates fear of failure and insecurity, so is good to use to help overcome low self-esteem, but also to encourage playfulness and childlike optimism. Not to be used when someone is overly confident or lacks boundaries.

Other keywords: motivator, childlike joy, happiness, laughter, release with optimism, letting go, openness to all that is.

Orange stones: carnelian, orange calcite, tangerine quartz, fire agate, fire opal, wulfenite.

Brown

Brown is earthy, fertile, capable of inspiration, a deep thinker, insecure, slow moving, but capable of supporting vast work and growth, the spring just before growth, the winter just before snow, that which is capable of coming into being under its own power, slow steady strength, power held in check, deep (though not unlimited) patience.

Other keywords: steady, supportive, strength.

Brown stones: aragonite, smoky quartz, agate, lodestone.

Yellow

Yellow strengthens the conscious mind and intellect. It initiates happiness and strengthens self-confidence. Use when a person is stressed, tense, or unclear about direction in life, but avoid for someone who can be intimidating or overwhelming.

Other keywords: life, strength, the sun, happiness, spring, air, the morning, clarity, sight, intellectual pursuits, the day, quick changing, abundance, growth, challenge, achievement, leadership, capability.

Yellow stones: amber, citrine, tiger's eye, sulfur, yellow fluorite.

Green

Green is the color of healing and balance. It is used to release the heart chakra of deep-seated envy, resentment, etc. It is said to attract prosperity and luck. Green is a color of nature and therefore seen as regenerating and rejuvenating. As it is in the center of the chakras it is seen also as a color of balance. Use green when you feel selfishness, jealousy, or heartache, but avoid using green with anyone suffering with a low boredom threshold or who lacks vitality.

Other keywords: fertility, growth, finance, the Green Man, jealousy, spring/summer, healing, peace, calm, contentment.

Green stones: green tourmaline, green calcite, malachite, emerald, aventurine, dioptase.

Pink

Pink represents unconditional love. It can release emotional pain, fostering self-love, peace, and joy. It attracts friendships and is a powerful color for sending love to another. Use pink when experiencing emotional pain or feeling emotionally shut down.

Other keywords: feminine, sweet, romantic, innocent.

Pink stones: rose quartz, rhodochrosite, kunzite, manganocalcite, morganite

Blue

Blue calms the emotions and promotes healing in general. Blue ensures truth and honesty and is seen as the peacemaker. It stimulates communication and understanding. This is the color that is often used to represent healing. Use it to generate calm when nervous and when you need to speak your truth. It should be avoided when someone is too detached, cold, or unemotional.

Other keywords: emotion, water, the West, intuition, divination, spirituality, connection, the Mother, calm, inner knowing.

Blue stones: celestite, angelite, lapis lazuli, sapphire, kyanite, barite, chrysocolla, amazonite.

Indigo

Indigo is linked to the brow chakra, which relates to intuition and inner thoughts. It is an expansive color that stimulates the mind to think creatively and can calm the "monkey mind" when used in meditation. Indigo encourages you to think outside the box and generates calm thought processes. It is an excellent color to use to find one's inner stillness, but should be used with care if someone is aloof and unsociable.

Indigo stones: azurite, tanzanite, iolite, lazulite, sapphire, sodalite.

Violet or purple

Violet is linked to spiritual enlightenment and awakening. It is linked with royalty, spirituality, and higher awareness. Use violet when you need inspiration or wish to stimulate spiritual connection.

Other keywords: meditation, mystical, enlightenment, insight—spiritual and personal.

Violet stones: amethyst, purple fluorite, sugilite, lepidolite, charoite.

Clear

Clear stones help you to access your intuition and spiritual nature. They enable you to see things from a higher perspective and encourage purification. Use these crystals or white-colored crystals such as snowy quartz or white agate as "all-rounders" that can be programmed effectively to carry the energies you require.

Other keywords: clarity, transparency, space.

Clear stones: clear quartz, Herkimer diamond, selenite, diamond, danburite, apophyllite, topaz.

Black

Black represents self-control and inner power. It is used to ground and connect us to the earth. It can help us see all possibilities. Black is a protective color. It promotes the use of intuition to reveal all. Use black when you feel you want to disconnect or withdraw, or feel in need of protection. Black is void of all color—opposite to white, which includes every color of the spectrum and so should not be used when someone is overly negative or disconnected from others.

Other keywords: darkness, the occult, power, shadow, the unseen, endings, introspection.

Black stones: obsidian, galena, hematite, jet, black tourmaline, magnetite.

HOW THE COLORS OF CRYSTALS ARE CREATED

The color of a crystal is brought about by three different factors:

- The chemical composition of the stone and in some cases the "impurity" of the chemical composition—for example, aventurine displays a shimmering silvery green sheen, which is a result of the fuchsite mica flakes it contains as inclusions.
- Defects in the crystal lattice that affect the way that the light passes through the crystal, modifying it by reflection, refraction, or diffraction.
- Interference of light—in other words, the way that the crystal reacts with light. When a stone absorbs all light frequencies, it will appear black; conversely, a white stone reflects the

entire color spectrum and doesn't absorb any light. Opaque or translucent crystals absorb light rays, which are slowed and bent or diffused (refracted or diffracted) according to the atomic arrangement within the crystals. The color of the crystal is dependent on how the atomic structure affects the light photons within the crystal. The slower frequencies appear red/orange, the faster frequencies appear blue/violet, while the medium frequencies appear yellow/green.

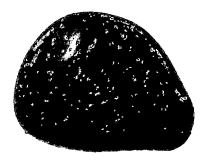

Reflection in an aventurine crystal

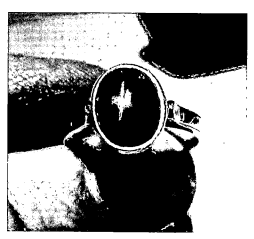

Star ruby, which exhibits pleochroism

Another factor that influences color is pleochroism—an optical phenomenon

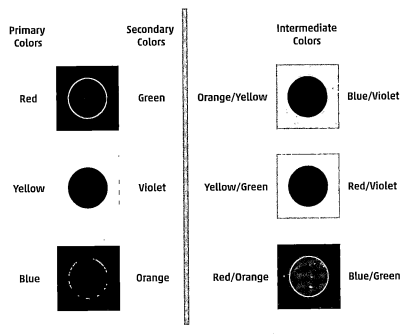

Primary Colors	Secondary Colors	Intermediate Colors	
Red	Green	Orange/Yellow	Blue/Violet
Yellow	Violet	Yellow/Green	Red/Violet
Blue	Orange	Red/Orange	Blue/Green

Examples of complementary colors

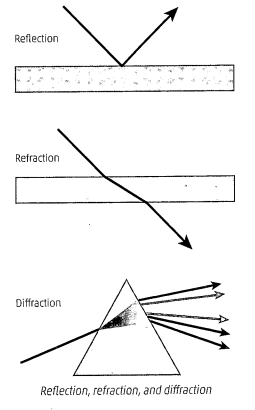

Reflection

Refraction

Diffraction

Reflection, refraction, and diffraction

that appears to give a crystal different colors when looked at from different angles. This commonly occurs with polarized light

Refraction can be illustrated by passing a laser beam through a transparent substance such as a crystal. The light enters the substance and slows down. It bends as it passes from air to substance. The light speeds up again as it leaves the substance, but the process has caused the light to bend, or refract.

When light from the sun or stars reaches the earth, it passes through air at about 300,000 km per second, but slows to 193,000 km/s when passing through quartz or 124,000 km/s through diamond. With each crystal type the speed at which light is processed varies.

So, crystals, due to their differing chemical compositions, formations, and so on, can filter certain parts of the spectrum and thereby release or hold on to certain colors. We can begin to see why color healers might regard crystals as "batteries" holding specific color energies.

QUICK QUIZ

What is the color of and the physical link to each of the seven chakras?

Color therapy can help to rebalance these energy centers by applying the appropriate color to the body and therefore realign, energize, or unblock the energy flow through the chakras.

CREATING A CRYSTAL MANDALA

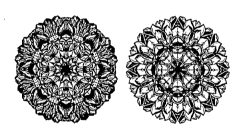

Mandalas

A mandala is a sacred space, often a circle that reveals some inner truth about you or the world around you. In Sanskrit, "mandala" means both circle and center, implying that it represents both the visible world outside of us (the circle) and the invisible one deep inside our minds and bodies.

A mandala can be used as a tool for meditation and can take any form, from a beautifully painted picture, Native American medicine wheel or dream catcher, to a simple pattern of pebbles on sand.

In the last century the Swiss psychologist Carl Jung developed the use of the mandala as an aid to psychological understanding. He drew a mandala every day to express his innermost thoughts and feelings. He felt that each drawing was individual and expressed a snapshot of his mental, emotional, and spiritual state of being. He considered that the images reflected his innermost self.

Jung believed that the top of the mandala indicated emotions that were held in the conscious mind, while the base symbolized areas of feelings and thoughts that were deep in the unconscious.

Reading the mandala is a way of connecting into our innermost thoughts and feelings. It may be elegant and intricate, or it may be simple and sparse. Try to understand the message of each symbol, shape, and color.

There is another guide to color correspondences that reflects color psychology—this may help to provide insight into your own mandala if you choose to copy and color in the mandala we have provided below. Appendix 4 at the back of the book also has a brief guide on how to interpret the mandala.

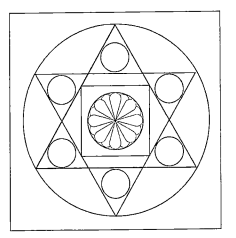

A blank mandala. There is a larger version of this image in appendix 4 that could be photocopied and colored in

QUESTIONS ON CHAPTER 4

1. Explain what a color wheel is and list the complementary colors as they appear on the wheel.
2. List the three different factors that influence the color of a crystal.
3. Explain what the electromagnetic spectrum illustrates.
4. Read two mandalas colored by different people. How accurate were they?

● ● ○ ● ◌ ●

CHAPTER 5

THE SUBTLE ENERGY SYSTEM

THE CHAKRA SYSTEM

Chakras are intersections within the body that link with the meridian systems and carry prana, chi, or life-force energy throughout the body. A way of visualizing them is to see the chakras as traffic circles and the energy lines as roads that flow in and out of the chakras.

Although we have seven major chakras, there are many more minor chakras contained in the body, such as in the palms of the hands, soles of the feet, tips of the fingers, and so on.

Chakras have been described by clairvoyants and yogis, who can see the energy field of the body, as spinning

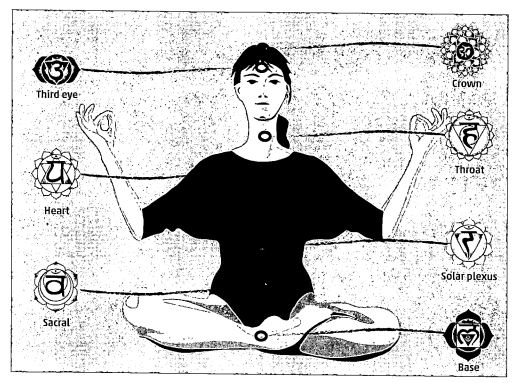

Positions of the chakras

wheels or vortexes of energy. The seven major chakras spin in alternate, opposite directions, taking in life-force energy and releasing this energy at the same time.

On a healthy person, these energy centers would be reasonably well balanced and aligned. Where there is an imbalance or misalignment, there may well be a physical manifestation of this as an illness. For this reason, healers tend to focus a great deal on providing the necessary energy to bring about balance, whether this be through spiritual healing, reiki, crystal healing, or some of the more conventional therapies, such as acupuncture.

It is important to note that these centers can be over-energized as well as under-energized. For most healers who do not have the benefit of clairvoyance, it is possible to use methods such as dowsing, muscle testing, intuition, or simply feeling the energy flow in order to determine where to direct healing energy.

Muscle testing was developed by Dr. George Goodheart, a trained chiropractor who also worked with acupuncture and other techniques relating to Chinese medicine. He treated the body holistically, viewing disease in the body as a disturbance of energy flow rather than just the physical representation that Western medicine treats. In using tools and techniques that relate to Chinese medicine, Goodheart explored a method of evaluating the state of the body by using biofeedback from muscles. Kinesiologists believe that stress that affects the energy flow and strains the body can be identified by a single muscle that presents as weakened when tested. Kinesiology practitioners work holistically and claim to identify physical, emotional, mental, and spiritual health issues using a range of muscle-testing techniques.

According to Ayurvedic tradition we all have a subtle body system that cannot (by most people) be seen, and throughout this system there flows a life-force energy. The seven main chakras are key points in the

Chakra Symbol	Name	Crystals
	Crown	Amethyst, Clear quartz, Diamond
	Third Eye	Sodalite, Lapis Lazuli, Sapphire
	Throat	Blue Lace Agate, Celestite, Aqua Aura, Blue Calcite
	Heart	Aventurine, Emerald, Moss Agate sometimes Rose quartz
	Solar Plexus	Citrine, Golden Tiger's eye, Amber
	Sacral	Carnelian, Orange Calcite, Topaz
	Base	Red Jasper, Ruby, Garnet

The chakras and their symbols

body that are said to relate to specific body functions, and when the flow is hindered or excessive this can trigger physical, mental, or emotional symptoms. It's possible to stimulate and balance chakras with crystals, and this can also be a powerful way of harnessing and shifting chakra energy to alter moods and enhance practices such as meditation or speaking.

A suggested, but by no means definitive, list of crystals that could be used to form a "chakra set" based on their color is the following:

Base: red jasper, ruby, garnet
Sacral: carnelian, orange calcite, topaz
Solar plexus: citrine, golden tiger's eye, amber
Heart: aventurine, emerald, moss agate, sometimes rose quartz
Throat: blue lace agate, celestite, aqua aura, blue calcite
Third eye: sodalite, lapis lazuli, sapphire
Crown: amethyst, clear quartz, diamond.

CHAKRA FUNCTIONS

Base chakra

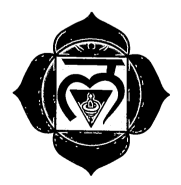

Base chakra

This is sometimes known as the root chakra, and in Sanskrit is *Muladhara*. It is the first major center and is situated at the base of the spine. It promotes the basic physical survival instinct. It is connected to materialism, courage, and vitality, and links us to the earth. Its traditional color is red, and it relates to the physical organs.

Possible symptoms of chakra dysfunction

Dysfunction of this chakra can lead to feelings of being unworthy, misunderstood, or unloved. It may lead people to be too materialistic, wanting more because of a lack of security. It can cause a dominant, intense survival instinct—perhaps because of not having been well looked after as a child, an experience from this lifetime or others. People may feel they don't want to be "here." Dysfunction is linked to problems with the legs, hips, and coccyx.

Sacral chakra

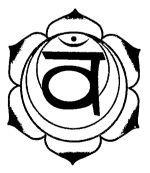

Sacral chakra

This chakra in Sanskrit is *Svadhisthana,* and it is also known as the navel chakra. It is the second major center and is situated approximately two inches (5 cm) below the navel. Its role is to generate sexual energies and creativity, to initiate new ideas, and to promote endurance, vitality, and strength. Its traditional color is orange, and it relates to the physical organs.

Possible symptoms of chakra dysfunction

Dysfunction of this chakra can lead to great difficulty in trusting, fear of being left alone, but also fear of loving. It can cause imbalances in sexual contact—frigidity or promiscuity, sexual dependency—or fear of or excessive desire for relationships, a tendency to be tense about sexuality, instability, drug addiction, a tendency to be addicted to anything—even love. Medical problems associated with dysfunction of this chakra include those of the large intestine.

Solar-plexus chakra

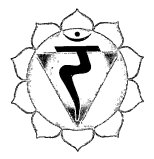

Solar-plexus chakra

In Sanskrit this is known as *Manipura*; it is the third major center and is found just above the belly button, below the ribcage. It relates to personal power, personality, and the ego, as well as being the energetic mouth of the body where life-force energy is taken in. The traditional color associated with this chakra

is yellow, and on the physical level it relates to the solar plexus area and the large intestine.

Possible symptoms of chakra dysfunction

Dysfunction of this chakra can lead to feelings of helplessness and weakness, allowing oneself to be controlled or trying to control and dominate others, showing off, struggling for success. People with dysfunction of the solar-plexus chakra may hold suppressed anger and suddenly express this through anger or rage, they may misuse their power, be aggressive or passive aggressive, and argumentative. Medical problems linked to dysfunction of this chakra include digestive problems, migraine, and immune-system difficulties.

Heart chakra

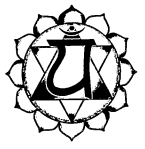

Heart chakra

This center, known in Sanskrit as *Anahata*, is the fourth major center and is found in the center of the chest, at the level of the heart. It relates to emotions such as compassion and love—ultimately to the promotion of unconditional love of the self and others. It is linked physically with the heart, thymus, circulatory system, cellular structure, and involuntary muscles (those that work automatically, without any need for conscious thought). There are two colors that are thought to relate to this center: pink and green.

Possible symptoms of chakra dysfunction

Dysfunction of this chakra can lead to feelings of loneliness, being lost, attention-seeking, feeling sad without a reason, guilt. A possible origin of such dysfunction is not having received enough love as a child. Dysfunction can also cause a tendency to exaggerate or to be over-caring of others, to take on the role of victim, to be constantly searching for new relationships, to feel depressed, repressed, or fearful of being oneself. Medical conditions linked to dysfunction of this chakra include asthma and air-based allergies such as hay fever.

Throat chakra

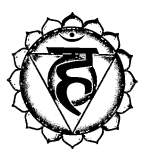

Throat chakra

The Sanskrit name for this center is *Visuddha*; it is the fifth major center and is situated at the base of the neck where the neck meets the clavicle and sternum. It is related to all aspects of communication. It is important to note that although this relates to making oneself understood by others, it also relates to us understanding others when they communicate with us. It also is linked to creativity, whether of the written word, painting, or talking. Physically, it can be linked with the thyroid, neck and shoulders, and the jaw. The color associated with this chakra is light blue.

Possible symptoms of chakra dysfunction

Dysfunction can lead to an inability to express oneself, difficulty with talking, singing, or movement. It can cause a person to have a tendency to speak harshly. Some believe that people with dysfunction of this chakra may have been punished in this or other lives for speaking their own truth, and might have been spiritual teachers in past lives. Dysfunction can also cause feelings of not being good enough, not being understood, a tendency to manipulate or lie, lack of clarity, and an inability to make up one's mind—this can also manifest in the solar plexus. This chakra can be blocked with unexpressed grief. Men may be more susceptible to blockages in this area when societal norms make it difficult for them to express their emotions. Medical problems of the thyroid and neck may be linked to dysfunction of the throat chakra.

Brow or third-eye chakra

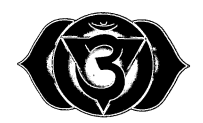

Brow chakra

This has the Sanskrit name of *Ajna*; it is the sixth major center and is sited in between the eyebrows. It is a center that is linked with clairvoyant and intuitive abilities, and many people seek to develop this chakra in order to achieve greater levels of psychic ability, such as clairvoyance or telepathy.

Physically, it relates to the cerebellum, nose, central nervous system, pituitary glands, and the left eye. The pineal and pituitary glands combine to help activate this center. Its color association is indigo.

Possible symptoms of chakra dysfunction

Dysfunction can lead to a person being very critical and judgmental, unhappy, and not convinced—nothing seeming to feel good enough. It can cause great difficulty in coping when intuition and logic struggle with each other, an inability to see links or patterns in things, and not wanting to look beyond the obvious.

Crown chakra

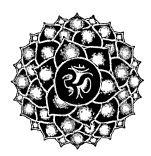

Crown chakra

Known in Sanskrit as *Sahasrara*, this is the seventh major center, located at the crown of the head. Its focus is thought to be our spiritual connection with God, the cosmos, or the universe. It empowers enlightenment, dynamic thought, and spirituality. Physically, it is linked with the cerebrum, the right eye, and the pineal gland. Colors related to this center are purple, white, and sometimes gold.

Possible symptoms of chakra dysfunction

Dysfunction can cause a disturbed connection with the divine and/or universal energy. This chakra is rarely "blocked" but often out of balance. This can manifest as delusion, illusion, being interested in only "spiritual" or "worldly" things and unable to cope with both. Conditions caused by disfunction include dyslexia, dyspraxia, and general coordination problems.

The chakras can work as pairs—for example, base and heart, throat and sacral, solar plexus and crown. Sometimes it is the balance between the two paired chakras that is the problem—one may be dominant, which can cause an imbalance. Once you correct one or the other of the pair they will come into balance.

THE CHAKRAS AND THE ENDOCRINE SYSTEM

The most complex and least understood body system is the endocrine system. This is made up of the endocrine glands and the hormones that they secrete—chemical "messengers" released into the bloodstream that regulate every function of the body.

Our hormones closely affect our emotions. Not very long ago it was thought that we

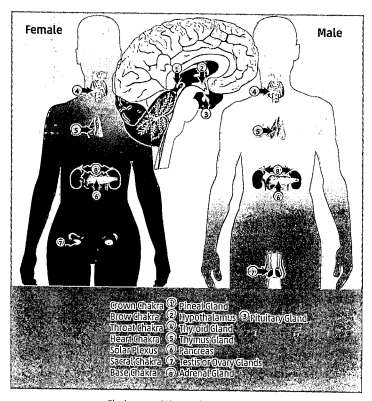

Female

Male

Crown Chakra ① Pineal Gland
Brow Chakra ② Hypothalamus ③ Pituitary Gland
Throat Chakra ④ Thyroid Gland
Heart Chakra ⑤ Thymus Gland
Solar Plexus ⑥ Pancreas
Sacral Chakra ⑦ Testis or Ovary Glands
Base Chakra ⑧ Adrenal Gland

Chakras and the endocrine system

had only around forty hormones circulating within the body; now scientists have identified nearly a hundred with specific functions, helping to maintain the fine balance of body functions by targeting specific receptor cells. Different hormones regulate different body functions— growth and maturation, blood pressure, metabolism, appetite and digestion, adaptation to stress, sexual response, reproduction, and aging are all delicately regulated by hormones.

Many Eastern religions link the endocrine system to that of the chakras, although this link is a subject of debate as there is some variation of opinion about which chakra is linked to which endocrine gland.

Here is a list of suggested links:

Chakra	Endocrine gland	Function
First—base, *Muladhara*	Adrenals	Excretion
Second—sacral, *Svadhisthana*	Ovaries/ testes	Reproduction
Third—solar plexus, *Manipura*	Pancreas	Digestion
Fourth—heart, *Anahata*	Thymus	Circulation
Fifth—throat, *Visuddha*	Thyroid/ parathyroid	Respiration
Sixth—third eye, *Ajna*	Pituitary	Cognition
Seventh—crown, *Sahasrara*	Pineal	Connection

Clearing blocks and imbalances

In order to clear blocks/imbalances, it is important to:

- understand why we have allowed them to be created in the first place
- not project guilt and blame onto others
- try to see what they have taught us
- ask, "Have I learned my lesson?"
- forgive—especially oneself.

Try to become conscious of negative thoughts and emotions. Know that it is possible to release them through understanding of the greater truth. Try to work from a position of unconditional love and compassion for yourself and others.

IMPORTANT NOTE: We must be very clear that if we are not qualified counsellors, anyone we work on should be encouraged to seek help from someone with the appropriate qualifications. However, it is possible to discuss issues with clients, and perhaps offer a perspective or viewpoint different to their own. The use of open-ended questioning—starting a question with "Who," "What," "Where," "Why," "When," and "How"—is usually an effective way of encouraging someone to open up.

CHAKRA SETS

Crystals can work beautifully as tools to balance the chakras. Choosing seven crystals—one for each major chakra—is an excellent way to provide a general tune-up during a healing session. However, the

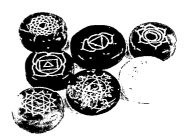

A chakra crystal set

combination chosen by the healer needs to be selected carefully. Many healers are guided by the traditional colors of the chakras and select crystals that represent the appropriate color of the chakra, such as:

Base—red jasper
Sacral—carnelian
Solar plexus—yellow tiger's eye
Heart—aventurine
Throat—blue lace agate
Third eye—sodalite
Crown—amethyst

An alternative is to consider using multicolored crystals—such as tourmaline, which is bi- or tricolored. Watermelon tourmaline has a pink center and a green outer ring. Would this color combination work with the heart chakra? Diamonds, clear quartz, and apophyllite hold the full spectrum of colors so may be good choices also.

Another point to remember is at what level you are working on the chakras. If, for example, you are working on a physical level, the quality of the chakra set may be "earthier" than if you were working on the chakras on a spiritual, emotional, or mental level.

A good basic chakra crystal set that will generally work effectively on all levels

CHOOSING YOUR OWN CHAKRA SET

Choose stones that you feel would be good for your own personal chakra set.

Suggested Crystal/Chakra List

Crown: amethyst, sugilite, charoite, tanzanite, fluorite, rutilated quartz, clear quartz, snowy quartz, citrine, white sapphire, white jade, lepidolite

Brow: sodalite, lapis lazuli, azurite, benitoite, sapphire, hematite, smoky quartz, tanzanite, iolite, labradorite, celestite, opal, amethyst

Throat: aquamarine, celestite, sapphire, topaz, turquoise, blue lace agate, blue quartz, chrysocolla, blue tiger's eye ("hawk's eye"), lapis lazuli, iolite, blue calcite, peacock ore, labradorite, spinel

Heart: green aventurine, amazonite, moonstone, unakite, apophyllite (white or green), peridot, prase, chrysoprase, emerald, aquamarine, green calcite, chrysocolla, dioptase, diopside, fluorite, jadeite, nephrite, malachite, green garnet, green apatite, rhodochrosite, rose quartz, morganite, watermelon tourmaline, alexandrite, kunzite and hiddenite, thulite (zoisite)

Solar plexus: citrine, yellow sapphire, amber, clear quartz, topaz, rutilated quartz, sulfur, pyrite (fool's gold), fluorite, desert rose

Sacral: carnelian, copper, orange calcite, dark citrine, topaz, orange jasper, tiger's eye, sunstone

Base: garnet, jasper, ruby, obsidian, tourmaline, smoky quartz, red tiger's eye, hematite.

consists of members of the quartz family—such as amethyst or clear quartz for the crown, sodalite for the brow, blue lace agate for the throat, rose quartz and aventurine for the heart, yellow jasper for the solar plexus, carnelian for the sacral, and red jasper for the base chakra—however, it is important to follow your own thoughts and feelings and choose a set intuitively.

Some crystal therapists feel that gemstone crystals—diamonds, rubies, sapphires, emeralds, topaz, and so on—emit a higher vibration and would serve as effective chakra crystals for working on a higher, more spiritual level with the chakras, but this can be very expensive!

Finally, another point of focus when selecting chakra sets is to consider the functions of the chakras and select stones that you feel support these roles. For example, rose quartz is generally considered to promote unconditional love—does this, therefore, make it a good choice for working with the heart center?

REIKI AND THE FOOT AND PALM CHAKRAS

Some other chakras that perhaps we don't often think about are, in fact, important to the effective practice of reiki. These are the foot chakras and the palm chakras.

The palm chakras are extremely important for those who engage in spiritual healing as they are a powerful tool for giving and receiving healing.

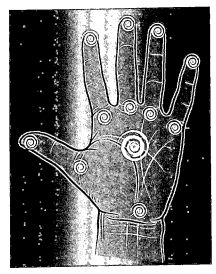

Palm chakras

There are seven chakras located in the palms—one in the middle of the palm, one at the wrist point, and another five in the fingers and thumb. The left-palm chakra rotates in a clockwise direction, whereas the right-palm chakra rotates in anticlockwise direction. It is said that left-palm chakras help receive energy, whereas right-palm chakras help sending and giving energy.

Your dominant hand sends out energy and your non-dominant hand receives. Someone with blocked palm chakras may find either that their energy scanning results are confusing or inaccurate, or that they cannot scan at all. For every reiki healer, it is extremely important to keep the palm chakras balanced as they emit energy, and the palms are used for scanning the aura.

Reiki functions of the palm chakras

- Healing oneself and others
- Scanning the aura
- Sending and receiving energy
- Helping to balance spiritual, mental, and emotional bodies
- Aiding and enhancing creativity
- Feeling the energy from crystals, healing, etc.

Underactive palm chakras lead to:

- illness
- an inability to receive
- an inability to accept healing
- hesitation in asking for help.

Overactive palm chakras cause:

- a desire to touch everything
- itchy palms
- rashes
- skin peeling
- an inability to let go; trying to hold on to issues
- compulsive shopping.

Techniques for opening/unblocking palm chakras

- Draw reiki symbols on your palms and cup them together, asking reiki to open the palm chakras.
- Draw reiki symbols on your palms. Imagine a red flower blooming in the middle of your palms. As this flower blooms, your palm chakras open.

- Ask your dowser to open and cleanse your palm chakras by holding the dowsing pendulum over them.
- Use a few grains of rock salt when you wash your hands.
- Practice making energy balls to activate the palm chakras.

Reiki functions of the foot chakras

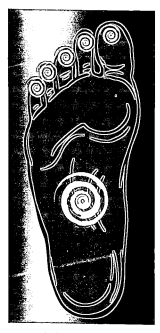

Chakras on the feet

- Manifestation
- Grounding
- Connection

We often forget to give reiki to the chakras in our feet while healing all the other major chakras. The foot chakras help pass divine energy to Mother Earth, which aids grounding and extends our energy into the earth.

Blocked or closed foot chakras can lead to:

- fatigue and tiredness
- insomnia and/or nightmares
- constantly feeling ungrounded
- feeling restless
- feeling disoriented and disconnected
- experiencing "slow healing" responses
- creativity blockage.

Healthy, functioning foot chakras:

- speed up the healing process
- make grounding powerful
- reduce tiredness and stress
- remove blockages related to manifestation
- heal insomnia and eliminate negative energies, psychic attacks, and nightmares.

How to open/unblock foot chakras

- Walk with bare feet on grass or on the ground.
- Imagine your foot chakras spinning and opening. Imagine roots coming out of your feet, grounding you deeply to Mother Earth. Imagine roots coming out of your feet and both chakras spinning and opening.
- Use grounding crystals to open the foot chakras. Example of grounding crystals are hematite, black tourmaline, Dalmatian jasper, and red jasper. Fill a tub or bucket with lukewarm water. Place some grounding crystals in the tub. Now place your feet in the water and

just play around with the crystals with your feet.

• Give reiki to your foot chakras.

INTERESTING INFORMATION

Tantric doctrine defines chakras as focus points for meditation. They are points within the body where nadis (see section "Nadis and the Kundalini" below) and meridians converge, and are also in places within the body where we experience emotions. They are storehouses of experiences and memories.

DISCOVERING THE CAUSE OF DISEASE

When trying to discover the cause of a disease, consider the following.

Physical body

How is the body reflecting a dysfunction? What are the implications? Perhaps a sore throat indicates an inability to communicate, too much talking, not enough listening, for example.

There may be a link to the chakra where the physical issue is situated.

Emotional/mental

When there are feelings of lack of self-worth, lack of self-love, lack of self-esteem, lack of self-expression, they might come from close personal relationships (parents?). This could be a sign of karmic issues that need to be considered—for example, are the parents the agents of karma?

Timing

When did the disease manifest? Some doctors are beginning to accept that cancer can sometimes be traced back to an emotional trauma or shock around two years prior to the disease manifesting.

Check what was happening at the time the disease became apparent. If the condition has manifested before, think about what was going on in that person's life at that time, and whether there is any correlation to the current manifestation of the illness.

Advantages/lessons of having the disease

An illness could be a sign that the person needs to make changes to his or her life but is resisting those changes. He or she might need to leave a job or relationship that is causing unhappiness, slow down, listen more, speak out more, and so on. Ask how the illness has changed the person's life and relationships.

If the condition is preventing the person from doing something, the key may be within this: what are the payoffs for having the illness? More attention? An ability to shirk responsibilities?

A NOTE ON DEATH AND DYING

When you work with someone who is dying, as a healer you are not working in order to bring about a healing in the conventional sense. The "healing" should support the process of dying, and this can be done in several ways:

• Giving the patient "permission" to die
• Centering the patient—freeing the patient of any fear of death he or she may have
• Providing a safe and pure space for the patient to pass on
• Being free of judgment
• Releasing any negativity/blocks from the patient's energy field
• Facilitating any decording (releasing energetically from others), and handing the patient over to guides, etc.

Familiar patterns

Do other family members or friends have a similar disease?

Spiritual evolution of the patient

Is the patient moving into a higher vibration and therefore releasing negative energy/energy blocks/releasing old patterns? This can manifest as flu symptoms, fevers, and upset stomachs, for example.

Tools that patients can use for themselves to help uncover the message of the illness include working with dreams, speaking to their higher self, or using visualization techniques. Bristol Cancer Care Centre uses visualization of a "Pac-Man" eating cancer cells, for example. Try to see the symbolism behind the disease. Ask for a symbol to counteract it.

THE NEW TRANSPERSONAL CHAKRAS

Below is a list of the latest chakras that many people are beginning to become aware of and work with. The suggested crystals should be placed near to the site of each chakra. It is easier if you are working on a couch—you will be able to place the crystals on the floor with the recipient lying on the couch, but otherwise place them as near as you can to the chakra site. You can dowse to check whether they are working by holding a pendulum over the area and asking for a simple *yes/no* answer as to whether the crystals are activating and strengthening the new energies. There are some suggested grid placements in appendix 2 at the back of the book, which indicate other ways you can work with these chakras.

The stellar gateway

This is the highest chakra at the current time, and located about twelve inches (30 cm) above the head. This chakra receives information from the divine. It acts as a filter for the information and energy to be received into the soul star chakra. Once open, the stellar gateway encourages us to experience unified oneness, wisdom, compassion, and constant connection to divine guidance. Its color is gold and so

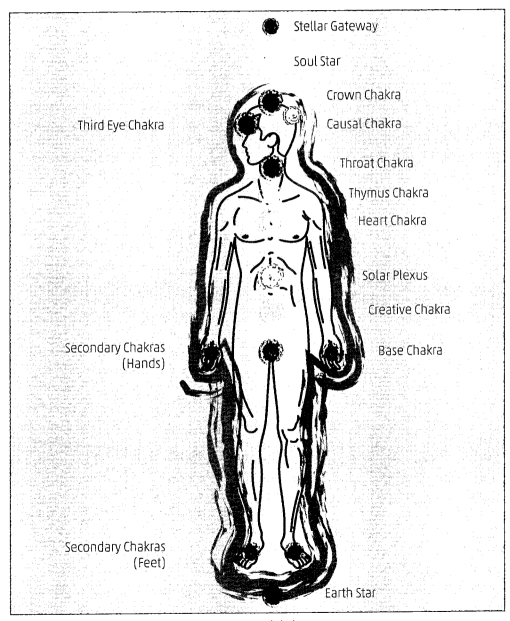

Stellar Gateway

Soul Star

Crown Chakra

Third Eye Chakra

Causal Chakra

Throat Chakra

Thymus Chakra

Heart Chakra

Solar Plexus

Creative Chakra

Secondary Chakras
(Hands)

Base Chakra

Secondary Chakras
(Feet)

Earth Star

Transpersonal chakras

crystals such as pyrite and peacock ore will work really well with this chakra, alongside angel aura quartz, or aura quartz, and garnet.

The soul star

Placed about six inches (15 cm) above the head, this chakra forms a bridge between the spiritual and the physical realms. Once activated, frequent attention to regular healing and psychic clearance is important to ensure a clear channel. You should try to ensure that you maintain a positive attitude to life and to those around you since your energy frequency (or vibration) may dip if you fall into negative outlooks and attitudes. This chakra helps to empower the focus of intention, whether this be for healing, manifestation, etc. Crystals for activating this chakra include snowy quartz, clear quartz, kyanite, selenite, and apophyllite.

The causal chakra

This chakra is situated in the center of the head, in the region of the pineal gland, three to four inches (7.5–10 cm) behind the crown. It receives energy from the soul star and filters it into the mental body (a layer in the aura). This chakra works to free us up from programmed belief systems, and regular meditation can help with this. When this chakra is activated it alters our perception and broadens horizons of consciousness. It can aid with keeping us in a state of calmness and groundedness. Crystals for activating this chakra include

aquamarine, white agate, lavender quartz, and aqua aura.

The thymus chakra

Located in between the heart and the throat chakra, this center is all about being able to "walk your talk" and say how you really feel, but combined with unconditional love. When this chakra is activated we learn that we can accept that everyone is different and we do not necessarily all have to agree, that we can express our thoughts and feelings honestly but also combined with love and compassion. Crystals for this chakra include turquoise and aqua aura quartz.

The earth star chakra

Located two to six inches (5–15 cm) below the feet, this chakra enables cosmic energy from the upper transpersonal chakras to be grounded and coherent. Crystals used for activating this chakra include shungite, black obsidian, and honey calcite.

Once all chakras are awakened and aligned, we are able to vibrate to a new higher frequency in line with the earth's new frequencies.

DIFFERING DIMENSIONAL STATES

You could argue that our changing brainwaves prove that we can inhabit differing dimensional states just by moving from one frequency to another (see brainwave-frequencies diagram).

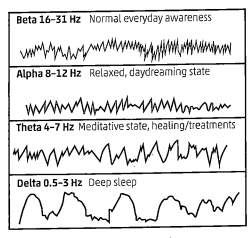

Beta 16–31 Hz	Normal everyday awareness
Alpha 8–12 Hz	Relaxed, daydreaming state
Theta 4–7 Hz	Meditative state, healing/treatments
Delta 0.5–3 Hz	Deep sleep

Brainwave frequencies

However, when we explore our spiritual reality it may be that we access other states of "being" or consciousness. These states are known as three-dimensional, four-dimensional, or five-dimensional states. Someone perceiving life through the third-dimensional state would perceive it very differently to someone experiencing life from a fifth-dimensional perspective. We probably all move from one state to another in a way that is like the fluctuations of our brainwaves, for example. The trick is to try to maintain as high a state of consciousness as you are able for as long a period as you can. Many people believe we will gradually leave the lower-dimensional states behind, and move into living within the higher dimensions. This is where connection to spirit is easier and more defined.

Third dimension

In this dimension, life is perceived from a purely physical state. Each person is an individual and there is no sense of interconnectedness. Your identity is tied into the material aspects of life—how you look, what you earn—fulfilment is tied to social status and making money, alongside a fear of lack or not having enough. Your thoughts have no power over your reality, and life is very superficial, with no desire to explore the deeper meaning to life. Although life can be joyful in this state, emotional pain can be difficult to manage. Within this state we rely only on the five physical senses of touch, taste, smell, hearing, and sight.

Fourth dimension

It is considered that the fourth dimensional state is a bridge between the third and fifth dimensional realities. In the fourth dimension we start to look for deeper meaning to our lives and explore our spiritualty. This suggests that our thoughts carry more power and can alter the reality we experience. Duality is still there, but with a greater sense of compassion and understanding as well as a growing sense of interconnectedness. Along with this comes a desire for a healthier lifestyle, meditation, an awareness of the effects of your actions upon the environment and others, and a quest to find your purpose and follow passions and to live a fulfilling and meaningful life. Along with the five senses we become aware of our sixth sense— ESP, or extrasensory perception—which includes intuition and aspects of spiritual connection.

Galactic

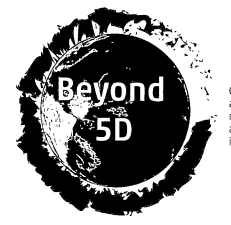

Currently this state of awareness can only be realized by body releasing and moving into spirit – i.e., dying.

Angels

Guides

Healing

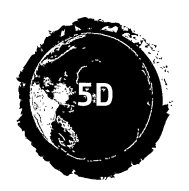

Stronger feelings of unconditional love and interconnectedness with others, planets and galaxies etc. Desire to live authentically, strong intuition. Each experience holds meaning.

EMF

Chakras

Higher chakras

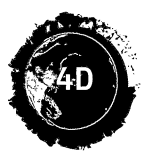

Awakening to something 'more'. Greater focus on the effects of your actions on others and the environment. Strong desire to find life purpose. Greater awareness of synchronistic events.

Fair health

Nutrition

Average health

Mental/emotional

Good health

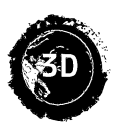

Viewing the physical state as all there is – no control over your reality. All your energies are invested in material wealth, etc.

The different states of being

Fifth dimension

Within the fifth dimensional state you accept that we are all one and that there is a higher purpose to life. Life becomes an adventure of growth, and experiences hold meaning and joy. There is a stronger feeling of love and compassion for all, with less judgment, as you understand that everyone's journey is individual to that person. You consider everyone equal and have the desire to live authentically and with integrity. Intuition is stronger, and you feel a connection to spiritual beings such as guides and angels, as well as the earth.

HIGHER STATES OF CONSCIOUSNESS

In higher states of consciousness, we lose perception of time and experience intense feelings of oneness. Our thoughts carry much more power and we have a very strong perception of the unity of consciousness. Time is no longer thought of as linear or measurable and instead feels limitless and immeasurable. Fear is no longer an emotion we experience and instead we live in a perpetual state of unconditional love. Currently many consider that to experience these states we have to leave our bodies behind, but others say that we can experience these states via near-death experiences, meditation, dreams, and even using certain plants or medicines.

It is believed that we are able to return our energy to the source, merge with others in our soul group, and travel to different galaxies, or reincarnate back to earth or other star systems. The soul is also enabled to evolve into a higher level of consciousness.

OTHER CHAKRA-CLEANSING TECHNIQUES

Wands are crystal tools that are often incorporated into massage and acupressure treatments. They are used to help create protective barriers, to direct specific energy, and to open and close the chakras.

1. Use a wand to pull debris from the chakra area that has built up over time—see it as clearing away calcified energy. Imagine the end of the wand as a crochet hook or suction pipe—start in the middle and work out, remember that the chakra flow is greater the further away from the body you are and it is important to check the direction of the energy flow of the chakra and work in this direction. Discharge the debris from the wand into the earth. When fully cleansed, overlay light into the gaps. Don't feel it necessary to cover every chakra with this technique—you may only need to do one or two.
2. Re-etch the chakra—this is a technique that can be used to repair the damage to the chakra system due to chemotherapy, drug abuse, and so on. Like the above technique, begin in the center with the wand and visualize a crystal "scaffold" being built. See the chakra being supported by this structure, allowing it to become more firmly anchored.
3. Infuse light into the center of the chakra. Hold the wand or crystal over the chakra

you wish to work on and gently tap the crystal, and at the same time visualize "drops" of crystal energy falling into the center of the chakra and infusing the chakra with the crystal energy.

CHAKRA IMBALANCES

Chakras may be out of balance for any number of reasons. In order to treat the imbalance effectively it may be necessary to identify possible reasons for it, which the recipient can address for the healing to be more effective. It is extremely important that the healer makes the recipient aware that he or she should also consider any mainstream treatment available, as crystal healing is a **complementary** therapy rather than an **alternative** therapy.

Bad diet, troubled relationships, stress, invasive treatments for ailments, drug and alcohol abuse, inappropriate spiritual connections—these are just a few of the life experiences open to all of us that can cause the chakras to become out of balance and alignment. This in turn can lead to dis-ease of the system, which ultimately can manifest in the physical as illness or disease. Mainstream medicine is now beginning to accept that cancer can sometimes be traced back to a trauma that occurred two or three years previously. The physical effects of stress upon the body are well documented, from increased blood pressure to nervous skin disorders. If you are to aid the patient to reach a point of balance and alignment there may be lifestyle changes that the patient needs to consider in addition to the healing offered.

It is important for the recipient to take responsibility for his or her own healing, and you should treat someone only with a therapy that you are qualified in.

NADIS AND THE KUNDALINI

Nadis are part of the Ayurvedic system of healing and are said to be linked to the autonomic nervous system (which controls body functions such as breathing, digestion, and heartbeat that are essential to life but not consciously directed). The word "nadi" comes from the Sanskrit *nad*, meaning "vibration" or "flow." Tantric texts tell us that there are over seventy-two thousand nadis contained in and around the human body, which direct prana throughout the body and auric field. As with the other systems to which they are linked—chakras and meridians—it is important for well-being that these channels can flow freely so that we remain vital and healthy. Hatha yoga is an effective tool in helping to maintain unhindered flow through these systems.

The chakras can be viewed as intersections, whereby the nadis carrying prana flow in and out of the chakras.

There are three main nadis, named "sushumna," "ida," and "pingala." All three of these start below the base chakra and their directional flow is alongside the seven main chakras. They all carry energy along the spinal column, with the pingala situated to the right of the sushumna, which runs centrally along the spine, and the ida placed to the left of the sushumna. Ida energy flow relates to lunar or feminine energy, which is

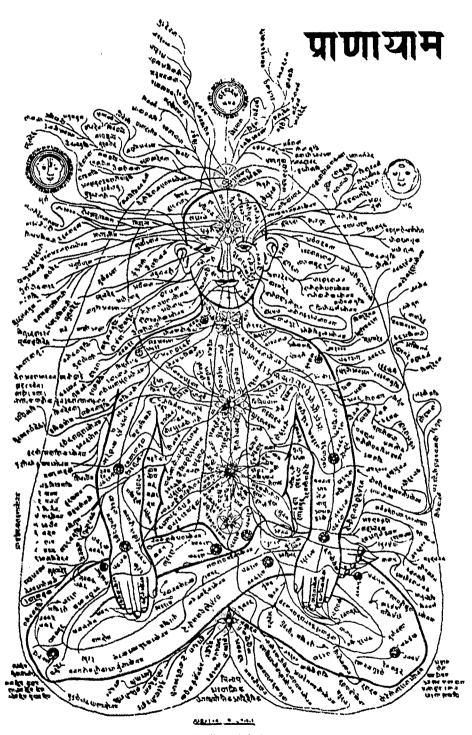

Nadis and chakras

sustaining and cleansing, whilst the pingala energy is identified as solar or masculine in type, which initiates and activates. All three of these main channels weave in between the chakras, meeting at the brow chakra.

Some people who work with vibrational energy refer to activating the kundalini, which is perceived as lying dormant at the base of the spine until stimulated by spiritual development or spiritual practices that activate "Shakti" energy, located at the crown chakra. This energy flows down the central channels and activates the dormant energy at the base of the spine. Once activated, all the energies unite and the individual is deemed to be enlightened. The kundalini is usually illustrated as a sleeping snake that rises through the sushumna channel, influencing each chakra as it reaches it. Movement of the kundalini is determined by the individual's spiritual and personal development, and it ultimately unites the ida and pingala, at which point an individual is balanced both in earthly and in spiritual matters and is truly at one with the universe.

This activation can occur "accidentally" through misuse of drugs, extreme-stress situations, and post-traumatic stress disorder, and can lead to mental imbalance. When this happens, it is best to withdraw from spiritual practices and anything that can stimulate this energy while the energies settle down. Grounding is especially important at a time like this. Thankfully this is a very unusual occurrence.

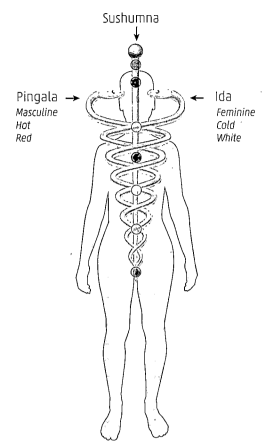

Ida, pingala, and sushumna

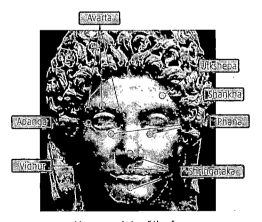

Marma points of the face

MARMA POINTS (VITAL POINTS)

Marma points are like Chinese acupuncture points and are also sometimes thought of as pressure points. Massage of the marma points stimulates electrochemical balance in the body. Small, gentle, circular movements by the finger on the points are thought to help release toxins from the body.

Marma points are the "junctions" where flesh, veins, arteries, tendons, and bones meet. When stimulated they ensure smooth functioning of the various bodily organs and systems. These junctions also form the points of vital life force, or prana.

They appear all over the body, and some consider them to be minor chakra points that aid the flow of prana energy. In martial arts, a warrior aims to hit these points specifically to disrupt the flow of prana, but therapists stimulate the same points in order to promote the energy flow. If a marma point in the leg is struck it can result in paralysis, or striking a point near the groin can result in impotency; to treat similar conditions, stimulation of these points such as with massage can aid the healing process.

There are 107 marma points in the body. Ayurvedic practitioners also believe that these points are where the pitta, kapha, and vata aspects connect in the body.

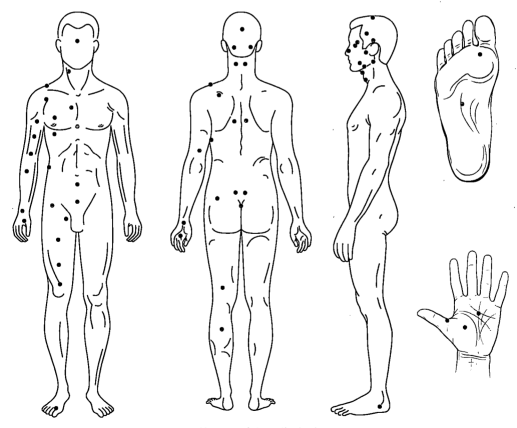

Marma points on the body

When working with Indian head massage, several of the points are stimulated, primarily in the eyebrow, sinus, temple, and ear areas.

Marma points are grouped according to the region of the body: there are twenty-two points on the arms, twenty-two points on the legs, three points on the abdomen, nine points on the chest, fourteen points on the back, and thirty-seven points on the head and neck.

QUESTIONS ON CHAPTER 5

1. Give a broad overview of each of the seven main chakras, including dysfunctions and correspondences. State which healing system uses chakras.
2. Use the chakra set layout and give your responses when receiving and the giving crystal therapy to others.
3. Explain what the transpersonal chakras are and give their names and placements.

● ● ○ ● ◌ ●

CHAPTER 6

MERIDIANS, AURAS, AND PROTECTION

WHAT ARE MERIDIANS?

● ● ● ● ● ● ◦ ◦ ◦ ● ● ● ● ◦ ◦ ◦ ● ● ●

Over five thousand years ago, the ancient Chinese identified twelve acupuncture meridians that linked to a specific organ of the body. Along these meridians they discovered an invisible nutritive energy, which they called "chi energy," that permeates all living things. This chi energy is the same as the prana, or life-force energy, that is the bedrock of India's Ayurvedic medicine system. Both acupuncture and Ayurvedic medicine are still practiced today and form the foundation for a growing array of complementary therapies, such as reflexology, reiki, shiatsu, and acupressure.

Practitioners of traditional Chinese medicine (TCM) believe that energy enters

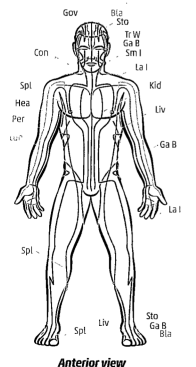

Gov   Bla
        Sto
        Tr W
        Ga B
Con   Sm I
        La I
Spl   Kid
Hea
Per   Liv
ʟυʔ
                    Ga B

                    La I

Spl

Spl
        Liv   Sto
    Spl   Ga B
                    Bla

Anterior view

The Body Meridians

Two Centreline Meridians:

Conception Vessel
Governing Vessel

Twelve Principle Meridians:

Stomach Meridian
Spleen Meridian

Heart Meridian
Small Intestine Meridian

Bladder Meridian
Kidney Meridian

Pericardium Meridian
Triple Burner Meridian

Gall Bladder Meridian
Liver Meridian

Lung Meridian
Large Intestine Meridian

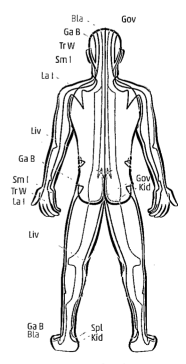

Bla   Gov
Ga B
Tr W
Sm I
La I

Liv

Ga B

Sm I   Gov
Tr W   Kid
La I

Liv

Ga B   Spl
Bla   Kid

Posterior view

the body through specific acupuncture points and flows to the organs, cells, and tissues, bringing a life-enhancing sustenance of chi/prana/life-force energy. This energy is found not just internally but externally, and with practice and awareness it is possible to assess and manage the energy flow. Commonly in TCM practitioners measure different pulses in the body and other bodily reactions to underpin the treatments and their effectiveness. TCM is also commonly coupled with herbal medicine.

Within Chinese medicine there are twelve pairs of meridians, as well as two other meridians that are known as "vessels" and carry the chi throughout the body, in

much the same way as veins and arteries carry blood around the body. The energy circulates the body in a twenty-four-hour cycle, and so at different times of the day there is more activity in one meridian than others.

Meridians are paired to reflect both sides of the body, giving twenty-four separate pathways, each related to a body organ, after which they are named. The twelve main (paired) meridians are:

- Lung (yin)
- Large intestine (yang)
- Stomach (yang)
- Spleen/pancreas (yin)
- Heart (yin)

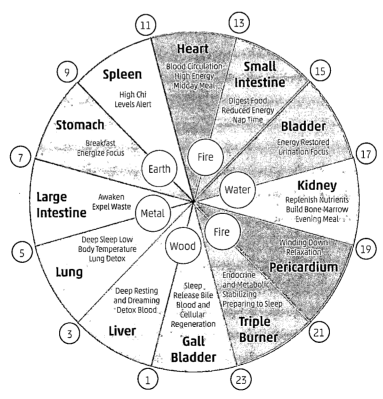

The meridian clock

Element	Wood	Fire	Earth	Metal	Water
Yin Organ	Liver	Heart	Spleen	Lungs	Kidneys
Yang Organ	Gall Bladder	Small Intestine	Stomach	Large Intestine	Bladder
Direction	East	South	Centre	West	North
Season	Spring	Summer	None	Autumn	Winter
Climate	Wind	Heat	Damp	Dry	Cold
Color	Green	Red	Yellow	White	Black
Sounds	Shouting	Laughing	Singing	Weeping	Groaning
Taste	Sour	Bitter	Sweet	Pungent	Salty
Orifice	Eyes	Tongue	Mouth	Nose	Ears
Sense	Vision	Speech	Taste	Smell	Hearing
Externals	Nails	Complexion	Lips	Body Hair	Head Hair
Sense Organs	Eyes	Tongue	Mouth / Lips	Nose	Ears
Tissue	Tendons / Nerves	Blood / Blood Vessels	Muscles / Flesh	Skin	Bones / Teeth
Emotions	Anger	Joy	Perseverance	Sadness	Fear
Planets	Jupiter	Mars	Saturn	Venus	Mercury
Developments	Birth	Growth	Transformation	Harvest	Storage
Activity	Walking	Watching	Sitting	Lying	Standing
Spirit	Spiritual Cosmos	Mental	Emotions	Physical	Will
Cycle	Birth	Growth	Maturity	Harvest	Rest

Meridian correspondences

- Small intestine (yang)
- Bladder (yang)
- Kidney (yin)
- Pericardium/heart constrictor (yin)
- Triple burner (yang)
- Gall bladder (yang)
- Liver (yin).

The organs that are linked to absorption and discharge, such as the stomach, gall bladder, small intestine, large intestine, and bladder, are yang (male) organs, while the organs that are blood-filled and regulate the body, such as the liver, kidneys, spleen, and lungs, are yin (female). The interaction between yin and yang meridians should in theory be in balance and create homeostasis within the body. It is when this is disrupted that illness can occur. Meridians are also classified as yin or yang according to the direction in which they flow, with yang flow down the body and yin flow up the body.

Thus, yin flows from the earth, running from feet to torso, as well as along the inside of the arms to the fingertips. In

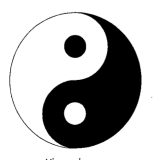

Yin and yang

addition to being perceived as feminine, keywords linked to the representation of yin energy include cold, wet, passive, gentle, dark, and negative. Yang flows from the sun and runs from the face to the feet or from the fingers to the face, representing masculine energy—other keywords associated with yang are positive, hot, dry, active, and strong.

Put another way, we can see that meridians have a positive and negative flow when working in synch with each other. In perfect circumstances this should be a continuous cycle, with each meridian's own characteristics performing specific functions for the organ that it is aligned to; however, with the stresses of modern-day life, this is not always the case.

ENERGY BLOCKAGES

An energy blockage is created when the energy flow between the twelve meridians is interrupted at any point and not able to flow freely, and this, as a result, can block chi, culminating in an under-energization in the remainder of the meridians. These blockages can be caused by an imbalance on a mental, physical, emotional, or spiritual level.

The basic belief of practitioners of TCM is that we are all born with the ability to heal ourselves of all physical ailments because we are chemically, organically, and mentally primed to survive. The role of chi energy is to connect each organ to the others so that they support any healing process taking place.

Two other meridians, known as the conception vessel and governing vessel, supply the chi energy to the front (anterior) and back (posterior) midline of the body.

Within a twenty-four-hour cycle, there are energy waves as each meridian (and its specific organ) receives an energy surge, followed by sedation when the energy surge passes.

TECHNIQUES FOR WORKING ON MERIDIANS

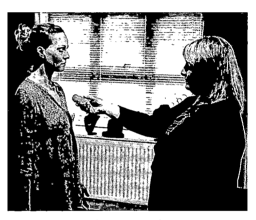

Working on meridians

1. This exercise can be carried out with the recipient either lying down or standing up. "Trace" a crystal point or wand in the correct directional flow of the energy. Try to sense any disruption to the flow, and either hold the wand at that place for a few moments or "remove" the blockage and discharge it from the point or wand into the earth, cleansing your crystal as you work. Then continue from the place you stopped at to the end of the meridian. You may need to trace the meridian a couple of times until the energy flow becomes smoother. You may

feel a "pull" or "obstruction"—this will be very subtle, and your sensitivity will increase as you practice. The recipient may well experience similar sensations as you work with the crystals.

2. Place crystals at each end of the meridian—check whether the crystals need to ground or absorb or balance the energy of the meridian before choosing the crystal. Ensure that you are aware at all times of the directional flow of the meridian, and if using points or wands take this into account when placing them. It is possible to use masking tape to fix the crystals in place if you wish.

CHINESE FIVE ELEMENTS

There are five elements that exist in TCM—fire, metal, earth, air, and water.

TCM practitioners believe that all of these elements are contained within us and that they influence our subtle energy system, which in turn affects our physical health. They see the five elements as part of a system where each element interacts with, supports, and controls the others.

Metal holds **water**—**water** helps to grow **wood**—**wood** is burned to create **fire**—**fire** burns every other element down into the **earth**—**metal** is extracted from the **earth**.

You can work out which element is most significant to you from your date of birth. The last digit of your birth year determines which is "your" element.

Russia leads in the recent and current research into the human energy field. Research in this area has been carried out

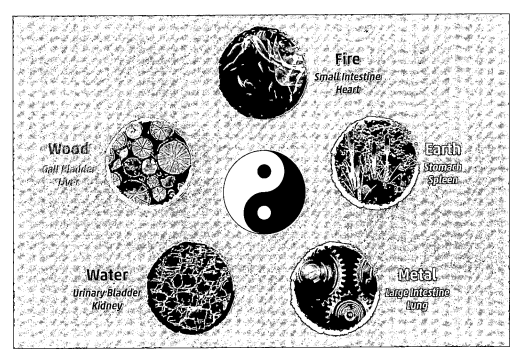

The five elements of traditional Chinese medicine

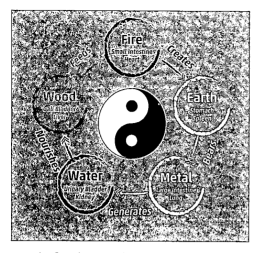

The five elements showing positive cycles

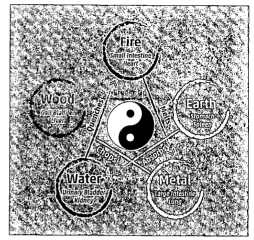

The five elements showing negative cycles

Last Digit of Birth Year	Significant Element	Suggested Crystals	Notes
0, 1	Metal	Pyrite, hematite, peacock ore	If your element is metal, you will have high standards and be the sort of person who prefers to live in a minimalist environment. You will be courageous, independent, and determined as well as ambitious. The downside is that metal-element people can be judgmental, uncommunicative, and dispassionate.
2, 3	Water	Blue calcite, blue lace agate	Those who are water elements are good diplomats and mediators. They can be persistent but are intuitive and flexible. They enjoy their own company but can also communicate with others and are perceived as quiet and peaceful, but at times can be overwhelming. They can find it hard to make decisions and suffer from anxiety.
4, 5	Wood	Mahogany jasper, Dalmatian jasper	Wood people are compassionate and generous. They can have good leadership qualities and are adaptable, but need to take care not to become overbearing or aggressive. When balanced they can be patient but also sensuous and are usually grounded individuals; however, if they are out of balance they will have a tendency towards aggressiveness and lack boundaries.
6, 7	Fire	Carnelian, citrine	Fire-element people have lots of energy, although it can be disorganized or chaotic. They tend to want to experiment and are adventurous, always seeking the next thrill. They have a passionate, creative, charismatic nature and can be warm, but in excess they can be destructive, impatient, and aggressive. They work well with wood people, who bring stability to a relationship between the two.
8, 9	Earth	Moss agate, jet	People connected with the earth element tend to be stable, patient, thoughtful, loyal, and honest. The downside for earth people is that they can be reserved and logical to the point of being "stick-in-the-muds." However, they are also empathic, nurturing, and responsible and can be the glue creating the bonds that enable things to hold together, as long as they don't become over-controlling or overprotective.

in Russia since the 1950s by Dr. Victor Inyushin at Kajakh University. His experiments suggest that the human body has an energy field that is composed of ions, free protons, and free electrons. Contained within the aura, or field, there is a balance of positive and negative particles, and if the balance is disturbed the overall health of the person can be affected. More recent research such as Lynne McTaggart describes in her book *The Field* comes from the area of quantum physics, and she has been credited with providing evidence-based research that has enabled a greater acceptance and understanding of the subtle energy system.

THE AURA

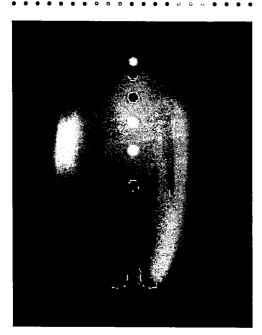

The aura

Charles Webster Leadbeater, a member of the Theosophical Society, published a book in 1910 called *The Inner Life*, where he described chakras as energy vortexes and the concept of auras as a field around the body. Later, Rudolf Steiner and Edgar Cayce interpreted further the Western concept of chakras and auras. More recently, authors such as Donna Eden and Barbara Ann Brennan have continued to develop our understanding of what they are and how they can be affected.

The aura is important for those using crystals because as soon as a crystal connects with our energy field it impacts on the subtle energy system, and usually the first contact is within the aura—such as when we pick up and hold a crystal, wear crystal jewelry, or use a crystal in a grid. Therefore, the aura has more effect on our health and well-being than the chakras do, as it is usually the first point of contact with energetic frequencies other than our own.

The aura contains within it the seven subtle bodies—these are a group of interconnected yet separate bodies that are the blueprints of the physical body and relate to our emotional, mental, physical, and spiritual states. Just as we can ascertain whether a chakra is out of balance, many people who are naturally psychic can pick up information from these fields, and many healers learn to process their perception of what is being held or manifested in the aura or energy field when they are carrying out a treatment. Most people agree that the energy field comprises seven layers, with the densest (or lowest frequency) being closest to the body and with each layer becoming finer (and higher frequency) as they are found further away from the body. Many people who see auras, however, don't perceive them around the body as seven layers; this is because of the continuous movement and interaction between each "body," which means the aura is usually defined as an amalgamation and is perceived as clouds of colors—some more dominant than others.

The aura has several functions:

• It works as a "sensor" around the body, both protecting and reading the energies from our environment as well as the energies generated by other people. Animals—especially dogs and cats—interact very sensitively on an auric level.

Rupert Sheldrake is renowned for his work in this area.

• The aura can act as an antenna, drawing positive energies into the energy field to nourish the energy system through the chakras and meridians. There is a growing understanding that walking in nature feeds the soul, while living in an urban environment can have the opposite effect!

• Just as the aura can act as an antenna for you to receive energy, it also sends out signals to others that provide information about you. Many people believe that the aura helps to attract both positive and negative energies to the

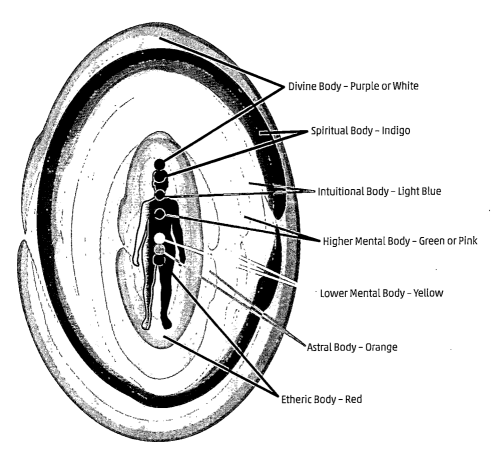

Divine Body – Purple or White

Spiritual Body – Indigo

Intuitional Body – Light Blue

Higher Mental Body – Green or Pink

Lower Mental Body – Yellow

Astral Body – Orange

Etheric Body – Red

Subtle bodies

individual, depending on what resonance is being given out by the individual through his or her aura.

Just like the chakras, each layer has its own correspondence. Below I have listed each subtle body along with its name and correspondence.

- The **etheric body** is the layer that is easily seen by most people and located nearest to the physical body. It can be detected by standing against a stark background and is perceived as a heat haze or "light" extending to around one to two inches (2.5–5 cm) away from the body. It is thought that this is the origin of the halos above the heads of figures portrayed in religious paintings. Its corresponding chakra is the **base**. The etheric body contains the etheric blueprint of the physical body, and so if a limb is lost, the "imprint" of the limb will remain in the etheric body. This may explain the "phantom-limb" syndrome whereby amputees often report sensations in a limb that no longer exists in the physical. One of the main aspects of this subtle body is that it is the gateway to the other energies held within the subtle energy system, and therefore is protective.
- The **astral body** is also known as the **emotional body** as emotional upsets, shock, and resulting trauma are held in this section of the energy field. Its related chakra is the **sacral**. This body holds the blueprint of our emotional and psychological stability within it, and is also affected by our sensitivity to those

around us. Sometimes this body is seen as separated into two layers, which relate to the mental and emotional aspects of us.

- The **lower mental body** is linked into the **solar plexus**. This is the thinking, or ego, part of the body and is still very much the center that the vast amount of humanity operates from (as opposed to the heart center, which is where we are now moving toward). Some clairvoyants report that they are aware of this body becoming brighter and radiating more when one is working with mental processes such as studying or writing. This is the level that would respond most to positive thought and affirmations.

These first three layers are connected to the personality within us. A lot of healers consider that it is within these three centers that many illnesses are based as they are the most closely linked with our physical being.

- The **higher mental body** is linked to the **heart** chakra, and at this point we start to relate to others, expressing love other than for the self, for example. Some healers maintain that past-life connections and trauma may be registered or held in this area. It is considered a bridge through which the lower energies pass into the higher energies and vice versa, and therefore there is a filtering or transformative role that this body fulfils. The positioning of this body extends to about six to twelve inches (15–30 cm) around the physical body.

- The **intuitional body**, sometimes called the etheric or **causal**, is connected to the **throat** chakra. In this body we are thought to hold the template or blueprint of our consciousness—in other words, the perfect form that we aspire to, or our spiritual template. It extends about twelve to twenty-four inches (30–60 cm) from the physical body.
- The **spiritual body** is linked to the **brow** center and connects us with higher spiritual awareness. It is through this center that we experience spiritual ecstasy—usually in combination with the heart chakra—and a closer connection with and realization of God. This body usually extends twenty-four to thirty inches (60–75 cm) from the physical body.
- The **divine body** is linked to the **crown** chakra and commonly accepted as connecting and allowing our divine consciousness to flow through us. Some claim that within this body is held past life, karmic, and other information on the soul. It is this body that reacts first to a request for protection and its outer edges are perceived as strong and resilient. It extends thirty to forty-four inches (75–110 cm) generally around the body.

It is important to understand that the subtle bodies are one of the first places where disease and imbalances can be perceived, and as these energy fields are extremely receptive to healing energy, it follows that we can help to prevent the manifestation of a physical illness or alleviate the presence of an illness by offering healing that helps to balance, realign, unblock, and re-empower the aura, and also the chakra system as the aura and chakras are interconnected.

To connect with the energy bodies, you can simply stand in front of someone and run your hands through his or her auric field, trying to detect changes in the density, temperature, texture, and so on, as you progress through each field. With practice you may be able to detect imbalances and areas where the field has become damaged.

Some healers work on the following approximations of distances of the subtle bodies from each other:

Subtle body 1—next to the physical body
Subtle body 2—1–3 inches (2.5–7.5 cm) away from the physical body
Subtle body 3—3–8 inches (7.5–20 cm) away from the physical body
Subtle body 4—6–12 inches (15–30 cm) away from the physical body
Subtle body 5—12–24 inches (30–60 cm) away from the physical body
Subtle body 6—24–30 inches (60–75 cm) away from the physical body
Subtle body 7—30–44 inches (75–110 cm) away from the physical body.

Although many diagrams illustrate the aura as a multilayered egg, this is misleading as it is perceived by many clairvoyants as energy fields that are multidimensional and that interpenetrate each other. These energy fields are constantly changing and shifting according to outside influences, such as those we encounter every day of our lives.

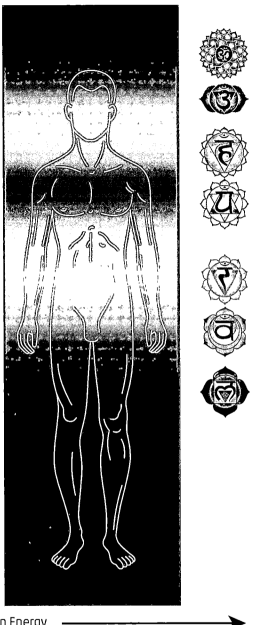

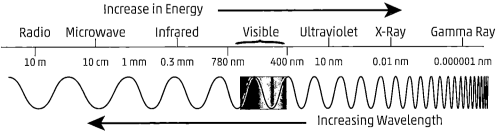

Electromagnetic spectrum in the chakra system

INTERESTING INFORMATION

Many energy workers believe that the aura can indicate potential illness through apparent energy imbalances in the subtle energy system—before the illness has been created in the physical body—and, if these are diagnosed quickly and treated energetically to redress the energetic imbalance, the physical manifestation of an ailment can be prevented.

"The Colors and shape of the aura are continually changing, influenced by not only physical health, but also emotions, relationships, the activity of the moment, the outer environment, etc." (Donna Eden of the Energy Medicine Institute).

"Illness is the result of imbalance. Imbalance is a result of forgetting who you are. Forgetting who you are creates thoughts and actions that lead to an unhealthy lifestyle and eventually to illness. ... Illness can thus be understood as a lesson you have given yourself to help you remember who you are" (Barbara Brennan, author of *Hands of Light*).

ELECTROMAGNETIC FREQUENCIES AND OTHER ENERGY STRESSORS

The electromagnetic spectrum within the aura is the radar for the physical body to emit coherent energetic information. If this field is not flowing, the vibrational frequency of the person will be below par. One of the fastest-growing sources of disruption to our energy fields is electromagnetic stress from man-made devices such as cell phones, microwaves, Wi-fi, and so on. Although a few years ago this was disregarded as something that wasn't really affecting us, there is growing evidence and acceptance that it is. With the advent of 5G the situation can only worsen. Currently, the World Health Organisation is investigating these effects, but things can only become more evident as we see an increase in radiation from cell phones, computers, smart meters, cars, and other electronic devices. Microwave exposure has proved fatal to animals in laboratory trials. Our bodies contain some crystal elements— such as calcite and salt—that respond to the ions generated through piezoelectrical charges, which have a neutralizing effect.

Reported symptoms of electromagnetic stress include:

* Fatigue
* Joint and muscle pain
* Decreased attention span
* Memory loss
* Difficulty focusing
* Insomnia.

Whilst keeping cell phones and Wi-fi routers out of your energy field as much as possible is a good idea, many people use shungite to protect themselves from electromagnetic frequencies. Avoid living near to a substation or near cell phone towers or power lines. Children will be more sensitive to these energies but also, as use of technology continues to grow, will be subjected to much more of these energies as they grow up.

Ways to alleviate electromagnetic stress

- Whenever possible, switch off or unplug electrical equipment and spend as little time as you can using a cell phone or working on a computer.
- Place a crystal—shungite, hematite, black tourmaline, lodestone—in or around the area.
- Bathe using a couple of handfuls of Epsom Salts and Himalayan sea salt or Dead Sea salt—just sit in a bath as hot as you can tolerate it and afterwards towel-dry off. (If you are pregnant, suffer from a chronic illness, or are a child, you should take medical advice first, however.)
- Have plants in close proximity to your computers and other generators of electromagnetic fields. Plants that have been proven—by NASA, no less—to absorb radiation include cacti, succulents such as stone rose, spider plant (*Chlorophytum comosum*), and mother-in-law's tongue (*Sansevieria*).

CRYSTALS AND BASIC FENG SHUI

The practice of feng shui is aimed at stimulating and protecting chi flow throughout your home or office. Feng shui practitioners believe that specific areas of your room, office, or house can have chi flow stagnated, just as we do in our physical bodies. A very simple way to stimulate the chi flow or luck in all aspects of your life is to place crystals in key areas of your abode. Here are some basic ideas to inspire you:

- **Near the entrance or front door** use obsidian, hematite, or black tourmaline. These crystals repel negative energies and offer amazing protection. They help to cleanse and purify the energy of the space but also the energies of everyone who passes through the front door.
- **In your office or wherever you frequently pay bills or work** use citrine and pyrite to stimulate abundance and prosperity in this area. Similarly, if you have a place where you leave bills and contracts, etc., you can place your crystals upon them to affect the same response.
- **In your bedroom** you can stimulate loving energies. The go-to crystal for this would be rose quartz; this can be even more accentuated if you choose a rose quartz that has been shaped into a heart. However, if what you want is really a good night's sleep, placing amethyst near or around your bed will help with this. Remember to program your amethyst to work when you want to sleep but to stop working when you want to wake up, or you might find it difficult to get out of bed in the morning!

A guide to placing crystal shapes in your home

Using crystals to balance and refine the chi energies circulating in your home or office is a simple practice that will ensure your personal spaces are as healthy and beneficial to you and your family as possible. Crystals generally will generate a strong earth elemental energy, but different formations will have different effects.

Clusters and geodes

Natural formations such as geodes and clusters work well and can be viewed as a statement piece or even art! The energy generated from a geode or cluster is generally very powerful—all those little points are sending out lots of individual positive energies directed outward like an explosion of chi; imagine the force of them combined! The most common type of crystal used for this is a clear quartz, but some people prefer to use amethyst geodes (sometimes known as cathedrals or caves) or apophyllite clusters.

Crystal towers or obelisks

Sometimes known as generators, crystals that are shaped like this tend to bring a grounding energy to the area they are placed in. This shape of crystal will bring a strong stabilizing energy to a room. A good place to put this shape of crystal is near a computer or in an office area of the room.

ENERGY PROTECTION
• • • • • • • • • • • • ·   · • • • •

Working with energy makes us more sensitive to the energy frequencies we draw to us, and so it becomes necessary to ensure that our energies are maintained and not compromised, which could lead to energy blockages or over-energy in any part of the subtle energy system, such as chakras and meridians.

Grounding and centering tools and techniques are the first things that anyone

should be aware of. Many people are confused between being grounded and centered. When you are grounded you are aware and focused on what is going on around you. You would probably be in alpha or possibly beta brainwave states (see diagram).

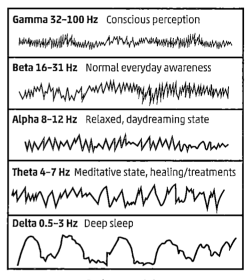

Brainwave states

When you centered you are calm and not stressed. I always describe being uncentered as feeling like you have had a shock, or being aware of adrenaline coursing around your body. Maintaining balance and equilibrium within your energy system promotes well-being and good health, and so it should be a priority for everyone who understands and works with energy.

Ensure that you have a balanced diet that is nutritious and healthy. Remember that food and drinks with caffeine and sugar can cause us to feel ungrounded and over- or under-energized. If this is what is happening to the physical body, then simply imagine how the subtle energy system is responding! Ensuring that we have the right balance of vitamins and minerals will support not only our physical body but also our entire energy system. If you want to make sure that you are getting the correct balance it is sensible to see a nutritional specialist rather than try to self-medicate with vitamin or mineral supplements. I have an acupuncturist whom I work with who ensures that my body receives the correct herbal concoctions for me as an individual, and I have never felt better. Also ensure that you are sufficiently hydrated, as this is often overlooked.

Be realistic about your shortcomings without beating yourself up. Knowing *and accepting* that you are usually someone who, for instance, would normally over-nurture others—a typical trait of a committed healer or therapist—means that you can recognize the warning signs and do something to minimize the unwanted extra work or responsibility.

Some seers say that time is speeding up. Life today certainly moves at a faster pace than it did years ago before the advent of technology. Instead of waiting for a letter, which may have taken two or three days to reach us, we now expect responses within moments of sending an email. This doesn't allow us time to reflect and consider our thoughts.

In our busy society there are more and more people suffering from anxiety and stress. Again, not something that is healthy for mind, body, or spirit.

I am sure that everyone reading this book can think of someone they know—possibly even a family member—who leaves them feeling drained. This is typical of what is known in esoteric circles as an "energy vampire." This not-very-nice term indicates someone whose level of prana or chi is low. The person usually is not aware that he or she has drawn energy from you, as it happens automatically, and probably just feels that after meeting or talking to you he or she is energized and more positive, while you may be feeling tired, demotivated, or even grumpy! It's on these occasions that wearing a crystal with protective qualities can help.

I always categorize energy protection at three levels:

- **Heavy-duty protection:** This is for when you are going into a difficult meeting where people are likely to be antagonistic, or when someone is actively wishing you harm. For this sort of situation, you could use strongly protective crystals such as black tourmaline. You can wear a piece of jewelry, hold a crystal, place some crystals on your desk (if at work), or have some in your pocket. This forms an effective barrier to repel any negative energies heading your way. However, for a working therapist who needs to build a rapport with clients this can prove to be too strong.
- **Boundary protection:** This is relevant when you are dealing with clients or members of your family or friends. It is gently supporting of your energy field while not having such a repelling effect on the other person. Carnelian is a wonderful crystal for this. It gently

supports boundaries without being obtrusive. Again, simply carry or wear the crystal.

- **Energy-raising protection:** This lifts your energy to a higher frequency and allows you to rise above petty irritations. Crystals you could use for this would be apophyllite, angelite, or selenite, but ensure that you don't become ungrounded in the process.

There are placements to clear stagnant/ negative energies in appendix 2 at the back of the book—once these have been done it is suggested that you select one of the above crystals and carry it around with you to maintain the benefits of the initial treatment.

Try to refrain from reading, watching, or listening to negative events and gossip— these activities lower your energy field's vibration but also that of the people they are directed against.

People are drawn to sacred sites to experience and work with the energies they generate. Sacred sites can be found all over the world. Some of the more well-known sites are Stonehenge and Avebury in the UK, the ancient pyramids of Giza in Egypt, the Mayan temples in Peru, and the River Ganges in India. If we accept that there are a positive and a negative to everything, it follows that where there are sites of human carnage—for example, Belsen, or battlefields—there will be an energy "echo" of the trauma that has taken place on that land. Therefore, when visiting such places, we may find that we are affected energetically—especially if we have had a

past-life experience at the site, should you accept that past lives are a reality, as do many longstanding religions. Sometimes visiting these sites can be a cathartic and healing experience, but other times we may need to clear the energies we have picked up from our visits there. Again, the grids in appendix 2 will help to clear anything like this from the energy field. However, if you feel that more help is required, work with a past-life regressionist or contact a healer or reputable psychic who can help you to understand and release any issues that have come up for you.

While many people who are working on an esoteric path acknowledge that there are angelic forces that align with and support us, we cannot accept this as a reality without also accepting that there may be discarnate energies—commonly, lost souls—who for one reason or another have not passed into the light and who can cause us harm. Even the Catholic Church acknowledges this reality as it is equipped to deal with similar forces through exorcism. The work involved in clearing these negative energies is specialized, and you should be well trained in order to work with them. Therefore, if you feel that you have encountered paranormal activity such as poltergeists or ghosts you should contact a specialist organization such as the Church. In the UK we also have the Spirit Release Forum—www.spiritrelease. org—which would be a good first place to contact and also offers full training with people who have had years of working within this specialist field. Spirit Release now offers all its courses online, so they are available to anyone anywhere in the world (see https://www.facebook.com/profile.

php?id=100057210140209). I am not trained or capable of fixing my car. If it is not working, I take it to a repair shop—it is the same for this type of work. When in doubt, contact an expert.

Here are a few coping strategies:

• Don't dismiss an instinct that you need to take protective measures. React to the feeling, even if it is as simple as bringing a crystal into your energy field. You can also call on your guides and angels for support and protection. Visualizing a shield of protection or a bubble of light around your aura also supports your energies. Intention is always a powerful tool if it is coupled with trust and belief.
• Keep your energies at the highest vibration possible. You can do this by playing uplifting music or watching a film that makes you laugh or stimulates joyful feelings within you. Also, refrain from overindulging in substances such as caffeine, which can boost your adrenals and cause anxiety, etc.
• Clear your energy field. You can do this simply with the visualization given above or any other visualization that appeals to you. You can also create a spray from spring water and Bach Rescue Remedy and spray into your aura. This will help clear the aura. If you are feeling positive you could also send similar energy to the perpetrator. It's an overused phrase, but sending love and light shouldn't always be reserved for those we care about. Often people with a more negative outlook on life and others need healing themselves.
• If possible, detach from people or places that make you feel negative—it is not weak to walk away from anything or anyone who doesn't make you feel as positive about yourself and your life as you can. In fact, it is a strength to recognize that there are people and places that no longer serve your best interests.

QUESTIONS ON CHAPTER 6

1. Explain what meridians are and from which healing system they are worked on.
2. Name the Chinese five elements and describe how they support and control each other.
3. Describe the aura and its functions; list the seven subtle bodies contained within it.
4. Explain why energy protection is important.

● ● ◉ ● ◌ ●

CHAPTER 7

MAKING YOUR OWN GEM ESSENCES

HISTORY OF GEM ESSENCES

Flower remedies are thought to have been used for centuries by various cultures, such as Australian Aborigines and Native American Indians. The Aborigines are said to have practiced a form of flower-essence therapy for thousands of years, involving ingesting flowers soaked in rainwater or sitting among inedible flowers, because they believed they could improve a person's well-being.

Probably the best-known flower remedies—those of Dr. Edward Bach—have been around since the 1930s. The remedies he developed, now known as the Bach (pronounced "batch") flower remedies, consist of thirty-eight plant- and flower-based remedies, which have each been

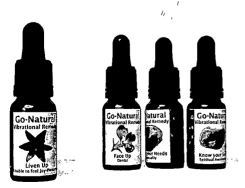

Flower and gem essences

devised to treat a different emotional state. The remedies are said to work by stimulating the body's capacity to heal itself by balancing out negative feelings.

Edward Bach was a well-respected Harley Street doctor practicing conventional medicine and homeopathy for many years before he turned his back on conventional medicine in favor of the healing properties of plants and flowers.

The process involves flowers being placed in water for about three hours at an appropriate time so that solarization can take place and the water becomes infused with the energy vibrations of the flowers. Once the water has been infused with the flowers' energy it is mixed fifty-fifty with brandy, creating what is known as the mother tincture. This is then further diluted with brandy to make the stock essence, which is the usual dilution to appear in the shops.

As the remedies are mixed with brandy, their shelf life is basically as long as the brandy stays good—usually around ten years. However, it is still important that the remedies are stored out of direct sunlight and away from heat sources.

In addition to the remedies themselves there are many other products that can incorporate flower remedies, such as aura sprays, made by using flower and gem essences in combination with essential oils. The growing popularity of these new products is due to an increasing awareness and acceptance of vibrational medicines and their positive effects on personal well-being and stress management.

Since the 1930s people in the West have used flower remedies, and although they haven't understood how they work, they have found them beneficial in releasing old emotional wounds or ties as well as for "emotional first aid"—Rescue Remedy is probably the Bach range of essences' bestseller and is made to support emergency emotional situations such as shock, but also to calm the nerves when one is being challenged by a job interview or examination, for example. Many actors acknowledge the use of Rescue Remedy to calm first-night nerves or stage fright.

If we accept that emotional balance and equilibrium are vital for our overall well-being, flower and gem essences or remedies are an important tool we can use to maintain our energy centers as well as bring them back into balance when life throws us challenges.

MAKING GEM ESSENCES

There are many ways to make a gem essence (flower remedies would be made in similar ways, but as this is a book on crystals, I will focus on making gem essences in this

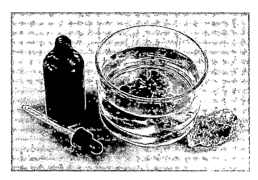
Making a gem essence

chapter). There are also several names that gem essences are known by—remedies, elixirs, and so on—these all mean the same thing: water that has been energized with crystals.

Commonly, gem essences are confused with essential oils and homeopathic remedies— they are neither of these. Essential oils are oils extracted from plants by a process of distillation, and homeopathic remedies are created using a process called succussion.

If you are intending to make a gem essence by immersing a crystal in water, remember when you are selecting the crystal to choose one that will not be damaged by this. Toxicity is another thing you need to be aware of—in the section "Toxic Crystals" below there is a list of crystals that could be poisonous if ingested or put on the skin.

Making a gem essence involves simply putting a crystal either in or near spring water. Incredible as this sounds, science is starting to recognize that water is a more complex material than we had thought. Professor Masaru Emoto has carried out experiments, which are well documented on the internet and in his books on the subject, whereby he discovered that the molecular structure of water could be affected by human consciousness, but also by flowers, crystals, sound, and intention.

The length of time the crystal needs to be near or in the water can vary, and if you are adept at dowsing this is a good way to check whether the gem essence is ready.

Putting a few drops of mother tincture into another bottle containing alcohol creates a "stock essence" that is the equivalent of the remedies and essences that can be bought in shops. In addition to the basic remedy, sometimes people will incorporate other energies such as moonlight/sunlight, reiki (including reiki symbols), sound, color, or the energy of a specific place or time.

Some people are averse to using alcohol, and instead water solutions can be preserved (preservation is the reason alcohol is incorporated into an essence) using vinegar or vegetable glycerin, although the essence is nearly always not so long-lasting or stable.

HOW YOU CAN USE YOUR GEM ESSENCES

- **Orally:** The most well-known and common way of taking remedies is to either place them straight on the tongue from a dropper or to add a few drops to water and sip it during the day.
- **For animals:** You can add a remedy to their drinking water, or if you have a cat or dog you can place some in the palm of your hand and stroke your pet with the remedy.
- **On the body:** You can add gem essences to bathwater, or you can rub them into pulse points or acupuncture points.
- **On energy points:** You can massage gem essence into chakras, marma points, acupressure points, meridian points, and so on. Place a drop on your finger and gently rub or massage the area.
- **In the aura:** To prepare an aura spray all you need is a clean spray bottle containing either spring water or perhaps a flower water (rose or lavender can be easily obtained from

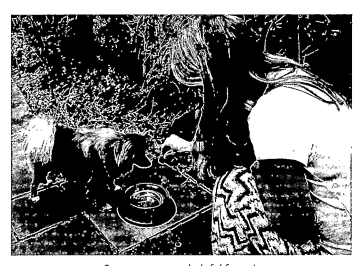

Gem essences are helpful for pets

RECIPE FOR AN ESSENTIAL-OIL ROOM SPRAY

As oil and water don't mix, you need to use something called an emulsifier, and there are a few different things you can use.

Ingredients:

Emulsifier—you can choose between witch hazel (about ¼ liter) and salt (Epsom salts, Himalayan salt or sea salt; you need around 1 tsp per ½ liter water)
Water
½-liter spray bottle
Around 10–15 drops of essential oil

Mix together the oil with the salt or witch hazel and stir or shake vigorously. Add water and give another shake. Add the water gradually until the smell seems right—if you add too much water you will have to add more oil.

Suggested mixes:

Calming: 5 drops of peppermint oil, 5 drops of lime oil, and 3 drops of spearmint oil
Relaxing: 5 drops of patchouli oil, 4 drops of lavender oil, and 2 drops of vetiver oil
Uplifting: 5 drops of grapefruit oil, 5 drops of orange oil, 4 drops of bergamot oil, and 2 drops of lemon oil

- **Adding to creams or lotions:** You can either make your own creams and lotions or you can get an inexpensive, unscented cream, lotion, or oil and mix the remedy into that. These can be incorporated into facial treatments, reflexology treatments, etc.
- **Setting energies:** You can add gem essences to a bowl of water with flowers floating on the top—this can be a lovely focal point in a room. You could also add an essence to an oil burner along with any essential oils you wish to burn to fragrance the room, but also to clear and create beneficial energies within the room.
- **Using on the ends of crystal wands, massage stones, and points:** You can empower a wand or crystal point by placing a drop of an essence on the end of the crystal.

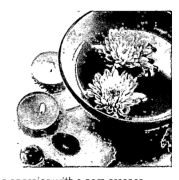

Setting energies with a gem essence

your local pharmacy). Add five to ten drops and spray into your aura. You could also use this as a room-clearing spray. You can be as creative as you like with this method—perhaps making a room-clearing spray or a grounding spray uplifting by choosing the relevant crystals and some aromatherapy oils as well. If you add a little alcohol, such as vodka, this will allow the essential oils to disperse. However, use your spray quickly as it will not last more than six to eight weeks.

TOXIC CRYSTALS

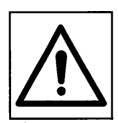

A word of warning: never immerse the following crystals in water to make a gem essence because of their potential toxicity. If you want to make an essence you can create it by placing the crystal **next to** the water, but never in it (I would also recommend using the essence only for "off-the-body" uses, such as room sprays). Please note this is not a definitive list—it just includes some of the more easily available crystals, so always check any crystal you intend to use.

Alexandrite—contains aluminum
Amazonite—contains copper
Aquamarine—contains aluminum

Azurite—contains copper
Beryl group—contains aluminum
- **Bixbite**
- **Emerald**
- **Aquamarine**
- **Goshenite**
- **Heliodor**
- **Morganite**
Black tourmaline—contains aluminum
Boji-stones (aka moqui balls, shaman stones, shamanic star stones)—contain some sulfur, pyrite, and/or marcasite
Cavansite—contains copper
Celestite—contains strontium
Chalcopyrite (peacock stone)—contains copper and sulfur
Chrysocolla—contains copper
Cinnabar—contains mercury
Copper—poisonous
Covellite—contains copper and sulfur
Cuprite—contains copper
Dioptase—contains copper
Dumortierite—contains aluminum
Emerald—contains aluminum
Fluorite—contains fluorine
Galena—contains lead
Garnet (spessartine, almandine, uvarovite, rhodolite, hessonite)—contains aluminum
Gem silica—contains copper
Hematite—will rust, but not toxic
Iolite—contains aluminum
Kunzite—contains aluminum
Labradorite—contains aluminum
Lapis lazuli—contains pyrite
Lepidolite—contains aluminum
Magnetite—will rust, but not toxic
Malachite—contains copper
Moldavite—contains aluminum oxide
Moonstone—contains aluminum

Morganite—contains aluminum

Pietersite—fibrous form contains asbestos

Prehnite—contains aluminum

Pyrite—contains sulfur

Ruby—contains aluminum

Sapphire—contains aluminum

Selenite—although not toxic, it is friable: tiny shards may break off in water

Serpentine—fibrous form contains asbestos

Smithsonite—may contain copper

Sodalite—contains aluminum

Spinel—contains aluminum

Spodumene (kunzite)—contains aluminum

Staurolite—contains aluminum

Stibnite—contains lead and antimony

Stilbite—contains aluminum

Sugilite—contains aluminum

Sulfur—poisonous

Sunstone—contains aluminum

Tanzanite (gem variety of zoisite)—contains aluminum

Tiger's eye—fibrous form contains asbestos

Topaz—contains aluminum

Tourmaline—contains aluminum

Turquoise—contains copper and aluminum

Vesuvianite—contains aluminum

Wavellite—contains aluminum

Wulfenite—contains lead and molybdenum

Zircon—contains zirconium, radioactive

Zoisite—contains aluminum

DISCERNING WHAT AN ESSENCE DOES

1. Take note of events that happened just before, during, or after the making.
2. Record the habitat, color, etc.

3. Using a pendulum or muscle test, ask the following questions (or any others that you think of):
   a. Which chakra does the essence mainly work on?
   b. Which chakras does it work on physically?
   c. Which ones does it work on emotionally?
   d. Which ones does it work on mentally?
   e. Which ones does it work on spiritually?
   f. Which subtle bodies does the essence work on?
   g. Which element(s) dominate in the essence?
   h. Which meridians does it affect?
   i. What results are obtained when working with core shamanism?
   j. Ask about any other thoughts, images, dreams, etc.

When you have dowsed/intuited these questions—and others you may come up with—you can start to put down any words that seem significant. Once you have gathered ideas, you can start to write a few sentences that will bring your notes together, taking note of repeating images or patterns.

Then you are ready to try your essences on a few sensitive friends!

MERIDIAN MASSAGE

This is a quick and simple technique that works well with gem essences. You can do it on yourself or on a partner.

- Place a couple of drops of one or two gem essences you've selected into your hands and rub your palms gently together.
- Keeping your hands a few centimeters off the body, start at the heart area and sweep down the inside of the left arm and up the outside of the same arm using a stroking motion.
- Repeat on the other side, starting opposite the heart and moving along the inner and then the outer arm.
- Go back to the heart area and gently sweep both hands from the heart over the face and head, and along the back as much as you are able.
- Finally, sweep the backs of the legs, up the inside of the legs, before returning to the heart area.

Repeat two or three times. You may wish to use a little more essence each time you cover a circuit or choose different essences for each repetition. Those who are sensitive to energies may be able to pick up where the energy feels slightly sticky or over-energized. Likewise, those receiving the massage may feel slight energy shifts as the essences help to regenerate and balance the meridians.

QUESTIONS ON CHAPTER 7

1. Explain what a gem essence is.
2. Name five toxic crystals and say why you should never immerse these crystals directly into water to make an essence.
3. Describe three ways you can use a gem essence.
4. Make two gem essences and record in a journal how you tested your essences for their qualities.

CHAPTER 8

ANIMAL HEALING

Although we humans can benefit from healing—or energy rebalancing, as I prefer to call it—it is just as beneficial for animals, and actually, for the sceptics among us, a fascinating example of how working with energy cannot simply be the placebo effect, for animals would not respond in the ways that they do if there were nothing more to it than that.

Although I don't have pets, I have been fortunate enough to experience some interesting reactions when giving healing to various dogs and other animals. In all cases the animal in question has approached me and sat or lain near to my hands. I have found that I don't need to move my hands, as the animal shuffles itself into the next position it wishes my hands to be placed upon, then becomes still until it senses it has had enough, and either moves on to the next position or walks away. However, as animals—like children—cannot communicate effectively with us there are several rules and regulations that anyone wishing to give healing to pets needs to abide by. The relevant acts are listed below.

RULES AND REGULATIONS

The laws relating to working with animals in the United States vary from state to state. In some states no one but a veterinary surgeon is allowed to work on an animal at all; in others it isn't even necessary to have veterinary approval to undertake therapeutic work such as crystal healing. So it isn't really possible to give any general guidelines—practitioners wishing to work with animals will need to check the laws and regulations in force in the state where they are working.

The situation in the United Kingdom is far simpler, and there are two main acts that practitioners working with animals need to be aware of.

The Veterinary Surgeons Act 1966

The Royal College of Veterinary Surgeons does accept the work of crystal therapists in providing the relief of suffering and does accept crystal healing as an acceptable alternative therapy.

Prior to treating an animal, you must ensure that the animal has been treated by a vet. You should have the permission of the owner. Healing should not be used as a substitute for veterinary treatment. You are not allowed to suggest a diagnosis. If healing is provided in the knowledge that veterinary advice has not been sought or taken it is considered an offense and can lead to prosecution under the 1966 Act.

The Animal Welfare Act 2006

The Animal Welfare Act 2006 confers a duty of care to animals—this means that anyone responsible for an animal must take reasonable steps to make sure the animal's needs are met. The person must look after the animal's welfare as well as ensure that it does not suffer, and this applies to all animals. Therefore, when providing alternative or complementary therapy, if you become aware that an animal needs veterinary treatment that it is not receiving you are obliged to urge the owner to seek veterinary advice as a matter of urgency. However, the administration of first aid in an emergency for the purposes of saving life or relieving pain is permissible.

BENEFITS OF GIVING HEALING TO ANIMALS

There are numerous benefits of giving healing to animals:

- It maintains and possibly improves your pet's well-being.
- It accelerates healing following surgery or illness.

- Reiki can provide pain relief and relaxation to facilitate and enhance the body's natural healing response.
- Healing stimulates connection and bonding between you and your pet.
- Promoting relaxation and stress reduction can help with behavior modification, especially with animals who have experienced abuse or suffer from anxiety or overexcitement.
- These issues can be exacerbated by stress, and healing modalities such as reiki have a calming effect on the pet and may help make it more receptive to training.
- Healing provides comfort for both the owner and the pet when an animal is undergoing traumatic events such as operations, or when it is dying.

INTERESTING INFORMATION

Hands-on healing with animals can really give you more confidence in the effects of healing. Animals tend to respond very well to treatments and often seem to be intuitively aware of what they need. In my experience, they approach me for healing and move away once they feel it has been completed. What I find so affirming about working with animals is that they cannot be affected by the placebo effect, but also they are unencumbered by doubt and fear of receiving a treatment so accept it unconditionally.

ANIMAL CHAKRAS

In previous chapters we have covered the human chakra system. Animals have a

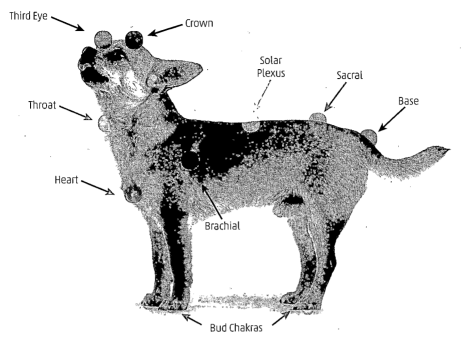

Third Eye • Crown

Solar Plexus • Sacral • Base

Throat • Heart • Brachial

Bud Chakras

Animal chakra points

similar system, with the addition of one other chakra. Their aura or energy field is usually wider than ours because they operate on a more sensory level than humans.

In addition to the above "main" chakras, there are minor chakras on all four paws and near the base of the ears.

Main animal-chakra correspondences and placements

Base chakra (Muladhara, *the first key chakra*)

Color: red.
Location: base of the tail.
Physical correspondences: adrenal glands, spine, bones, legs, colon, anus, kidneys, tail, and back paws.
Attributes: survival instincts; vitality and grounding imbalances will surface as fear or anger, constipation, and issues with paws and legs.
Suggested crystals: hematite, red jasper, brecciated jasper.

Sacral chakra (Svadhisthana, *the second key chakra*)

Hematite   Red jasper   Brecciated jasper

Amber   Moonstone   Carnelian

Color: orange.

Location: above the sex organs on the stomach.

Physical correspondences: pelvis, reproductive organs, genitals, small and large intestines, stomach.

Attributes: desire, creative energy, sexual energy, sensory pleasures. Imbalances can manifest as sexual dysfunction, jealousy, etc. Animals with severe dysfunction can also experience back pain, or bladder or elimination problems.

Crystals: amber, moonstone, carnelian.

Solar plexus chakra (Manipura, *the third key chakra*)

Tiger's eye   Citrine   Pyrite

Color: yellow.

Location: upper chest, a few inches back from the front legs.

Physical correspondences: stomach, pancreas, gall bladder, liver, kidneys, diaphragm, nervous system, lumbar vertebrae.

Attributes: ego, determination, assertion, equilibrium. When imbalanced can result in excessive fear or aggression. Poor digestion can sometimes indicate imbalances on this chakra.

Crystals: tiger's eye, citrine, pyrite.

Heart chakra (Anahata, *the fourth key chakra*)

Malachite   Aventurine   Rose quartz

Color: green.

Location: the heart area and chest.

Physical correspondences: heart, blood and circulatory system, lower lungs, chest, immune system, thoracic vertebrae.

Attributes: unconditional love, forgiveness, and compassion. Imbalance may result in the animal experiencing anger or showing hostility. It may also develop heart-related problems. This can affect the animal's ability to experience or express love.

Crystals: malachite, aventurine, and rose quartz.

Throat chakra (Visuddha, *the fifth key chakra*)

Turquoise   Blue quartz   Blue lace agate

Color: light blue.

Location: the upper throat area.

Physical correspondences: thyroid, lungs, respiratory system, throat, mouth, vocal cords, forelegs, and paws.

Attributes: self-expression and communication. Imbalances can be detected through frustration, excessive barking, etc.
Crystals: turquoise, blue quartz, blue lace agate.

Brow chakra (Ajna, the sixth key chakra)

Sodalite   Lapis lazuli   Amethyst

Color: indigo.
Location: between the eyes and a few inches higher up than in humans.
Physical correspondences: left hemisphere of brain, left eye, base of skull, nervous system, side of head, forehead, nose, ears.
Attributes: intuition, imagination, vision, focus, and concentration. When imbalanced, coordination and balance can be affected.
Crystals: sodalite, lapis lazuli, amethyst (note: if amethyst is used for the brow chakra, usually clear quartz is selected for the crown).

Crown chakra (Sahasrara, the seventh key chakra)

Amethyst   Snowy quartz   Clear quartz

Color: purple, white, or gold.
Location: top of the head.
Physical correspondences: right hemisphere of brain, right eye, cranium, cerebral cortex, side of face.
Attributes: inner wisdom, spiritual nature, universal connection. Imbalances may result in depression, lack of enthusiasm, and lethargy.
Crystals: amethyst, snowy quartz, clear quartz.

Brachial chakra (the eighth key chakra)

Animals have an eighth chakra, referred to as the brachial chakra, that humans do not have. It is the main energy center in all animals and links directly to all the other chakras. When performing any healing work on an animal it is recommended to begin with the brachial chakra.

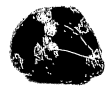 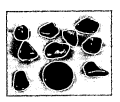

Snowflake obsidian   Onyx

Color: black.
Location: either side of the body, in the shoulder area.
Physical correspondences: none.
Attributes: This is the center that governs the animal-human interaction, and where the animal-human bond is formed and carried. When out of balance, pets may be timid and fearful. Alternatively, they could be aggressive when approached and shun human connection.
Crystals: snowflake obsidian, onyx.

TECHNIQUES FOR WORKING WITH ANIMALS

Crystals can be used in the following ways, but do take care that your pet is not able to eat or swallow crystals.

- Put a tumble stone on its collar. There are specialist dog tags with crystals connected to them that you can purchase.
- Make a gem essence and put it in your pet's water bowl, or alternatively place some of the essence on your hand and stroke it into your pet's fur.
- Spray a gem essence in your pet's bed by putting a few drops of the gem essence into a mister, or, even easier, you could simply place a crystal tumble stone such as rose quartz in the mister and mist any area where your pet sits or lies, such as its bed.
- Holding a crystal in your hand, gently stroke your pet with the crystal—this works well if you combine the crystal you use with a relevant chakra as shown above.
- Set up a distant-healing grid of crystals that can't be reached by your animal, which you can "send" to your pet.

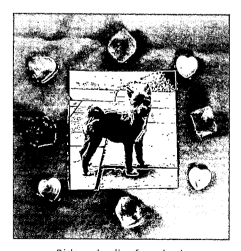

Distance healing for animals

INTERESTING INFORMATION

Rupert Sheldrake is a scientist who has carried out extensive research on something called morphic resonance. One of the most common examples of this is the telepathy exhibited by dogs and cats when they show signs of anticipating when their owner is returning home or when they are going to be fed, taken for a walk, and so on. Although these reactions from the pet could be taken as coincidence or routine expectations, Rupert Sheldrake has conducted many experiments that have proved otherwise. His most well-known case study was with an adopted dog named Jaytee. For more information, take a look at his website (www.sheldrake.org), or read his book *Dogs That Know When Their Owners Are Coming Home.*

While you are healing an animal:

- Observe any changes in the animal's body language or temperament.
- Notice the healing energy coming through your hands—this is particularly relevant for those trained in reiki or other spiritual-healing techniques.
- If you are working on a large pet, you will be able to move your hands from one position to another. Smaller pets such as gerbils or mice can be healed, using cupped hands, in one go. Any animals deemed to be dangerous should be given distance healing.
- Try to be sensitive to the animal's feelings and approach it with love and open-heartedness. Place your hands just

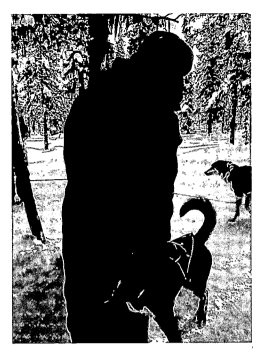

Healing an animal

above the animal rather than physically touching, unless you and the pet are comfortable with closer contact. Stay in the same position for several minutes and be guided by your pet's movements. When you do move your hands, ensure that you do so slowly and gently, without sudden movements. Be aware that it is very common for animals to adjust their position to receive the healing coming from your hands.

- Gauge your animal's responses to the healing; it should appear relaxed and somewhat soporific.
- Be guided by your pet when to stop. Animals are very responsive to healing but also to when they have had enough. They often get up and just walk away.

QUESTIONS ON CHAPTER 8

1. Name the two Acts that practitioners working in the UK should be aware of if they wish to provide healing to animals, and explain their relevance.
2. Give three benefits for giving healing to animals.
3. Describe and name the eighth chakra, which is specific to animals only.
4. Suggest three ways you can use crystals to help your animal's well-being.

CHAPTER 9

● ● ◠ ● ˌ ●

CRYSTALS AND ASTROLOGY

Historically, astrology can be traced back as far as the Babylonian civilization; however, there is also evidence that shows that the ancient Egyptians, Romans, and Greeks also used astrology to make sense of their existence on the planet. We also know that it was widely used in Europe during the medieval and Renaissance eras.

In India crystals and astrology are strongly linked with the Ayurvedic system of healing, and interwoven into some religious beliefs, with the first mention of astronomical concepts being traced back to the Vedas (religious writings), from around 1000 BC. Large observatories were built at several locations in India to look at and help interpret the heavens—those surviving today date from the eighteenth century, but at some sites, particularly Ujjain, there are believed to have been very much earlier observatories.

Maharaja Sawai Jai Singh (1688–1744) built a new capital at Jaipur so that he could construct the observatory shown in the picture. The astronomy here is medieval, and makes no distinction between astronomy and astrology, yet the instruments are very futuristic and very accurate.

Although historically astronomy and astrology were linked—astrology is based on how the planets appear to move around the earth when observed from earth, whilst astronomy is the study of the stars, planets, and space—there is no longer the connection that there once was. The general modern view is that astrology is not science based, while astronomy is.

Even today many people use astrology to guide them through life. In India, marriages are arranged according to the astrological charts of the bride and groom, and the most auspicious date for the wedding is determined by reading the charts.

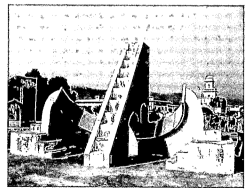

Sawai Jai Singh's observatory at Jaipur

Astrologers can draw up charts according to the focus and reasons for the person requesting them—here are some different examples:

- **Birth or natal charts** explore the idea that an individual's personality, life path, talents, and traits are determined by the time, place, and date of birth.
- **Horary charts** are an ancient form of astrology whereby the astrologer tries to answer questions by creating a horoscope for the exact time when a question was received and understood by the astrologer.
- **Psychological astrology** is connected to humanistic and transpersonal psychology.
- **Financial charts** forecast the movement of stocks, shares, and commodities in line with the movement of the planets.
- **Electional astrology** assesses the most auspicious time for specific events.

As we have already said, many ancient civilizations—India, China, Egypt, the Mayans, and the Incas—sought guidance from the stars and planets. In Europe, the ancient Greek, Roman, Celtic, and Germanic civilizations had systems of astrology. The wise ancients would look at the stars to determine times when it would be fruitful to plant the fields, or when it was the best time to get married, and so on. Even today there many gardeners and professional agriculturists who look to the movement of the moon to guide when to plant and when to harvest (see https://uk.rhythmofnature.net/gardener-calendar, https://permaculturenews.org/2015/01/26/moon-planting-guide/ and https://oldmooresalmanac.com/planting-by-the-moon/)—not such a strange concept when you accept that, as Isaac Newton established, sea tides are affected by the gravitational pull of the moon. In much the

same way, this pull affects the water content of the soil and when there is a full moon there is increased moisture, which encourages the seeds to grow.

Astrology is linked with medicine through the Chinese I Ching and Vedic astrology, which is linked to Ayurvedic medicine. In Europe the Western astrological traditions link with pagan customs.

Astrologers acknowledge that the lunar cycles influence our bodies and emotions. It's not such a weird concept if you think about it. Our bodies consist of around 75% water and if a full moon can affect the ocean waves why would it not affect us? Many people find it harder to sleep during a full moon, for example. The BBC reported that the police in Brighton in the UK were fielding more police officers during the full moon after research carried out in 2007 indicated that there were more violent incidents occurring at this time. A Brighton inspector, Andy Parr, said, "on full moons, we do seem to get people with ... stranger behavior—more fractious, argumentative."*

The practice of gardening and agriculture by the cycles of the moon is regaining popularity. The earth has a gravitational field that is affected by both solar and lunar cycles, and as the moon pulls tides in the seas it also causes moisture to rise in the earth. A new moon is the most advantageous time to plant, and half-moon or waning moon is the best time to harvest.

---

*"Crackdown on Lunar-Fuelled Crime," BBC News, June 5, 2007, http://news.bbc.co.uk/1/hi/england/southern_counties/6723911.stm.

BIRTHSTONES

Birthstones are commonly worn by both men and women in India, with the correspondences going back as far as 1000–2000 BC. The places the crystals are worn are deemed important too. (Some Ayurvedic practitioners believe each finger has a correspondence and that denotes where a ring should be worn: Jupiter—index finger; Saturn—middle finger; sun, moon, and Mars—ring finger; Mercury—little finger.)

Selecting your birthstone can be confusing as there are many different ideas about which stones correspond to which months.

Apart from the Ayurvedic list of birthstones shown in the chart, there are many other cultures and civilizations that have harnessed crystals to align with astrology and other healing systems, such as the North American Indians and Chinese astrologers. There are various cultures worldwide who have attributed healing properties to various minerals and crystals, also considering them to be the bringers of good and bad luck, as well as having the power to ward off evil or provide power, strength, or other correspondences. Gemstones such as diamonds, rubies, and sapphires were considered more powerful because of their clarity and rarity.

However, in 1912 the American National Retail Jeweler's Association created a new list of birthstones (see figure), adapting it in 1938 (by adding citrine), and again in 1952. The association maintained that the origins of its system could be traced back to Moses, who in the Bible talks about the "Breastplate of Judgement," which contained twelve gems, each engraved with the name of one of the twelve tribes of Israel. An alternate

Month	Birthstone		Month	Birthstone	
January	Garnet		July	Ruby	
February	Amethyst		August	Sapphire	
March	Bloodstone		September	Moonstone	
April	Diamond		October	Opal	
May	Agate		November	Blue Topaz	
June	Pearl		December	Ruby	

Ayurvedic birthstones chart

theory is that in the Book of Revelation, New Jerusalem was given twelve gems as "foundation stones," and these gems were used to signify the succession of birthstones for each month.

In 1937 the British National Association of Goldsmiths followed the American idea and adopted its own official list of birthstones, also by calendar month, which is still in use in the UK today (see figure).

Month	1912 American National Retail Jeweler's Association		1937 British National Association of Goldsmiths	
January	Garnet		Garnet	
February	Amethyst		Amethyst or bloodstone	
March	Aquamarine		Aquamarine	
April	Diamond		Diamond or Clear Quartz	
May	Emerald		Emerald or Chrysoprase	
June	Pearl or Moonstone		Pearl or Moonstone	
July	Ruby		Ruby, Carnelian or Onyx	
August	Peridot		Peridot or Sardonyx	
September	Sapphire		Sapphire or Lapis Lazuli	
October	Pink Tourmaline or Opal		Pink Tourmaline or Opal	
November	Citrine or Yellow Topaz		Citrine or Blue Topaz	
December	Blue Topaz or Turquoise		Turquoise	

UK and US birthstone lists

This explains the confusion that has grown up around which is the right birthstone for each month, compounded by the fact that different types of astrological correspondences don't follow neatly from one month to the next. When in doubt go with what intuitively feels right for you.

Date	Sign	Symbols		Keywords
21/3 - 19/4	Aries	♈ Ram		I want
20/4 - 20/5	Taurus	♉ Bull		I build
21/5 - 20/6	Gemini	♊ Twins		I communicate
21/6 - 22/7	Cancer	♋ Crab		I create
23/7 - 22/8	Leo	♌ Lion		I am
23/8 - 22/9	Virgo	♍ Virgin		I organize
23/9 - 22/10	Libra	♎ Scales		I relate
23/10 - 21/11	Scorpio	♏ Scorpion		I regenerate
22/11 - 21/12	Sagittarius	♐ Archer		I discover / explore
22/12 - 19/1	Capricorn	♑ Goat		I achieve
20/1 - 18/2	Aquarius	♒ Water Bearer		I evolve
19/2 - 20/3	Pisces	♓ Fishes		I imagine

The twelve signs of the zodiac

NATAL (BIRTH) CHARTS

The information required to draw up a natal chart is the date, time, and place of birth. From this information astrologers can look back and see how the planets would have been positioned at that precise point in time. As in astrology it is considered that the planets move around the earth, and therefore around you, the chart is shown from the perspective of you as the center.

A natal chart is made up of the following components:

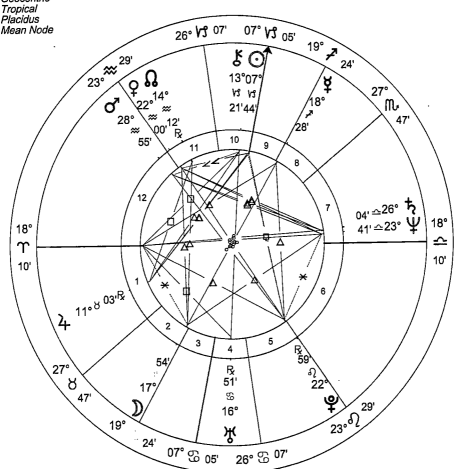

Transits 29 Dec 1952
Event Chart
29 Dec 1952, Mon
12:00 UT +0:00
london, United Kingdom
51°N30' 000°W10'
Geocentric
Tropical
Placidus
Mean Node

A birth chart

The **zodiac** represents the path the sun seems to take as it moves around the earth. It is divided into twelve sections—**zodiac signs**—each describing a distinct basic personality type. Each sign has positive and negative correspondences, with the hidden qualities of each sign known as the shadow, which reflects the negative side of the sign. For example, Taurus and Scorpio can both be jealous and resentful, while Gemini can be less than truthful. Being aware of both your positive and negative aspects can aid personal and spiritual evolution.

The **elements** represent the different ways that we experience and see life, and include **water**—sensing through emotions, **earth**—experiencing the world through the physical senses, **air**—connecting with life through reason, logic, and thought, and **fire**—intuition and knowing. Some charts have a balance of all of these elements, but in others they can vary considerably. Signs that share the same element—such as Aries, Leo, and Sagittarius, which are all fire signs—usually find that they resonate well with each other.

The **qualities** influence what a person's general approach is to life—whether he or she goes with the flow or likes order and structure, for example.

The **planets** and their placements are what make each chart individual, as the planets are continually moving and coming in and out of a chart. Some planets take longer than others to move in this way. They are forces that create events both in individuals' lives and also within the world.

The **angles** illustrate the progression through life, with the **ascendant** showing the soul at the point of incarnation or birth, and the progression through childhood, work, relationships, and so on.

The **houses** indicate areas of life that allow us to work with and experience the energies from the planets.

The **aspects** denote the connections between planets—a bit like an interconnecting web. When planets come together there is inevitably a chain reaction, and aspects can provide insight as to how these reactions will play out. "Easy" aspects show the planetary energies flowing more easily, while "hard" aspects can illustrate conflict.

Although the birthstones can relate to the star sign in a chart, crystal therapists can link the energies of crystals to a specific planet. This means that we can work with crystals to enhance or reduce the effects of planetary action at a given time, when a planet might be, for example, retrograde. (When a planet is retrograde it indicates potential delays or disruption, or might signal a time to wait and reflect. So, for example, if Mercury is retrograde, communications and plans can sometimes be stalled.)

A birth chart can help us understand every area of our life, including relationships, life paths, gifts, challenges, spirituality, and so on. There are many astrologers who specialize in specific aspects of astrology, such as business, medical issues,

Day	Planet	Symbol	Crystal Colour	Gemstone
Sunday	Sun	☉	Red	Ruby
Monday	Moon	☽	Orange	Pearl
Tuesday	Mars	♂	Yellow	Coral
Wednesday	Mercury	☿	Green	Emerald
Thursday	Jupiter	♃	Light Blue	Yellow Sapphire
Friday	Venus	♀	Indigo	Diamond
Saturday	Saturn	♄	Violet	Blue Sapphire

Astrological traits

or relationships. I have used astrology personally when I have felt that I have lost direction or when I needed guidance. I have also requested charts for my children at key points in their lives, to provide insight. Whenever I buy a christening gift, as long as the parents are happy for me to do so, I usually commission a chart for the new being on the planet. So far, every parent who has received one has found it to be amazingly accurate. It is a tool that provides new parents with insight into the child, which can be reassuring, insightful, and helpful in supporting their child's growth and development by pinpointing areas where the child may need encouragement, as well as gifts and talents that could otherwise go unnoticed or untapped.

INTERESTING INFORMATION

Nostradamus was a famous French astrologer, physician, and seer who authored a book of poetic quatrains (poems consisting of four lines) predicting future events that was published in 1555 and is still in print today. It is famous for a whole range of predictions that have come true, such as the Great Fire of London and the French Revolution, as well as more modern-day occurrences such as World War II and the assassination of President Kennedy.

USING ASTROLOGY TO EMPOWER A CRYSTAL TREATMENT

The twelve zodiac signs are divided into four groups, with each group representing an element (earth, air, fire, or water). Astrologers believe that your personality is influenced by the element your sign is in:

Water signs: Cancer, Scorpio, and Pisces
Earth signs: Capricorn, Taurus, and Virgo
Air signs: Aquarius, Gemini, and Libra
Fire signs: Leo, Aries, and Sagittarius.

Discerning your moon sign can help uncover the hidden, or "shadow," side of your personality. This can help us to work on deep-seated issues or emotions that we may not even be aware of.

The moon governs feelings and emotions and can represent the family, particularly the Mother qualities of the sign it occupies at any given time. It can influence the way we feel and respond to life.

There are many sites on the internet that can tell you what your moon sign is and its correspondences. Armed with this knowledge you can choose crystals that offer supportive or clearing energies, as appropriate.

Similarly, you could also work with the sun sign, which represents who we are and what we identify with. It is our creative individuality.

Each zodiac sign represents a particular characteristics in a person, which have both positive and negative aspects. The signs are can be grouped together in several ways:

- By element: **Fire** signs (Aries, Leo, Sagittarius) represent tendencies to be open to change, enthusiastic, and have leadership qualities. **Earth** signs (Taurus, Virgo, Capricorn) are practical and focus on achieving material goals and aspirations. **Air** signs (Gemini, Libra, Aquarius) are more intellectual and like to explore concepts, while **water** signs (Cancer, Scorpio, and Pisces) can be sensitive and emotional.
- Astrology further subdivides the signs into **cardinal, fixed,** or **mutable,** which indicate degrees of whether a person is open to change, movement, etc.
- Signs are also allocated a **masculine** or **feminine** bias; for example, Aquarius is a fixed air sign that is masculine, and an Aquarian personality would present with talents or life qualities relating to the intellect, individuality, tolerance, and connection to humanity. On the other hand, Virgo is a mutable earth sign with feminine aspects, so Virgos will have talents or life qualities of kindness, introversion, conservativeness, shyness, and skepticism.

One way to work with crystals and astrology is to create a **crystal grid**, which could represent a planet your chart indicates could be supporting or hindering you at a specific time. For example, Saturn Return (when Saturn returns to the position it was in when you were born) comes up for everyone at least twice in their lifetime as it normally occurs every twenty-eight to twenty-nine years. Some people can sail through a

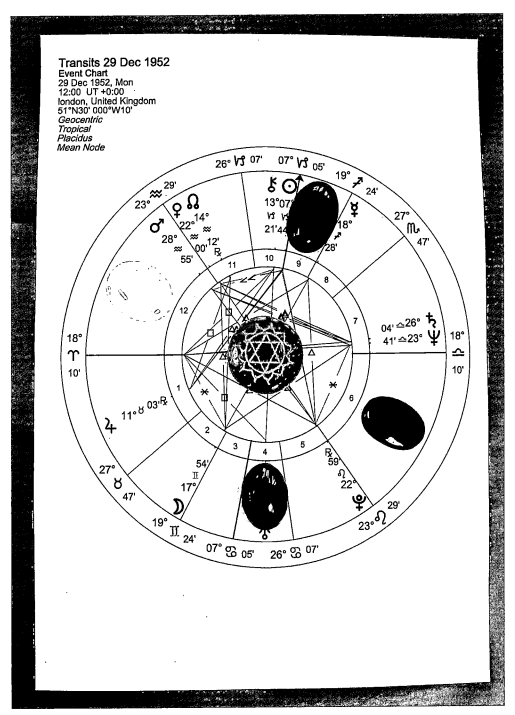

Transits 29 Dec 1952
Event Chart
29 Dec 1952, Mon
12:00 UT +0:00
london, United Kingdom
51°N30' 000°W10'
Geocentric
Tropical
Placidus
Mean Node

Using astrology to empower a crystal treatment

Saturn Return period, but for others it can bring life-changing events or period of introspection and reassessment. Astrologers believe that Saturn transits encourage us to take responsibility for ourselves and our lives thus far, so they can be challenging and life-changing but also life-enhancing—supporting us to leave behind what no longer serves us but also to acknowledge what we have and can achieve.

I would look at working with the crystal relating to the planet in the birth chart illustrated—in this case, Saturn is linked to blue sapphire. I would place this in a grid along with other crystals relating to how the person receiving the grid is feeling. If the person feels "all over the place" I would perhaps add some grounding crystals. If he or she feels a lack of motivation, I might select energizing crystals. For clarity it might be clear quartz. Or I might use a combination of all four, which would include the blue sapphire representing the planet itself.

There are also twelve houses in each astrological chart, and each house acts as a focus-finder, indicating the area of life in which planetary energies operate. For example, the first house represents individuality, which includes life, body, breath, physical appearance, and health. The second house represents personal resources, money, manner of living, and possessions. The fifth house represents creative endeavors, children, sex, and good fortune. So, if a client was blocked in her creativity, then it would be possible to work on that by placing crystals on a copy of her chart to help bring out the creativity and remove the block.

Pauline Gerosa is highly skilled in many aspects of astrology, and I have found her readings help almost as a route map that informs, motivates, and supports me when life doesn't seem to be running smoothly. Always ensure that your astrologer has been properly trained and that you feel comfortable with him or her. With knowledge of your date, time, and place of birth, your astrologer can draw up a chart for you with a written report of its interpretation. Or he or she might arrange a face-to-face meeting with you or, more commonly nowadays, talk with you by Skype, so that you can ask questions and discuss your chart and how to interpret it.

CRYSTAL RITUALS FOR WINTER AND SUMMER SOLSTICES

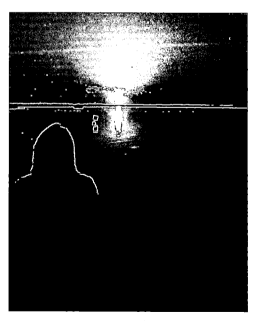

Summer solstice

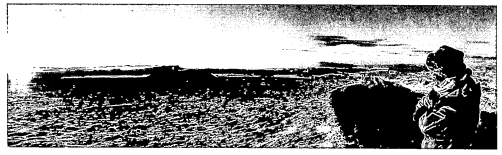

Winter solstice

Each year on June 20–21, the first day of summer (summer solstice) is marked by the earth tilting closest to the sun. In the northern hemisphere, this heralds the longest day of the year. On or around December 21, the winter solstice is the shortest day of the year. Astrologically, the winter solstice marks the start of the cardinal zodiac sign of Capricorn, while the summer solstice signals the sign of Cancer. Once the winter solstice has passed each day then has longer and longer periods of daylight, and so it is seen as a celebration of rebirth of the planet.

You can mark both solstices by placing items—preferably from nature, such as leaves and flowers—relating to that time of year on an altar, along with crystals that you feel support the energies:

Suggested crystals for summer solstice: citrine, sunstone, rutilated quartz, pyrite, carnelian, garnet.
Suggested crystals for winter solstice: moonstone, fluorite, amethyst, selenite, rose quartz, chrysocolla, labradorite.

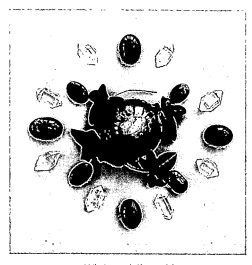

Winter solstice grid

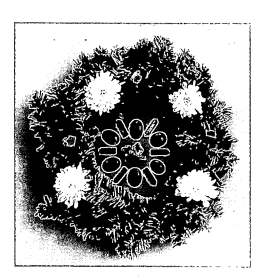

Summer solstice grid

Here are some rituals you can use to mark the summer and winter solstices, as well as some suggested crystals to use around those times.

Summer solstice

This is a time for connecting with the energies of the divine masculine.

Place the chosen crystals in front of you, creating your own mandala pattern with them. Choose an intention for the ritual—it may be to connect with the divine masculine energy force; it could be to manifest something, or simply to immerse yourself in the positive, activating energies of the season. Relax and breathe while you sit and meditate for around ten to fifteen minutes, holding the focus that you will be immersed in the codes of light that are generated at this time of year. When you are ready, breathe deeply once or twice and bring your focus back into the room.

Winter solstice

This is the time of year we go into hibernation mode. It is seen as a time for connecting to divine feminine energies.

Light a candle to illuminate the darkness. Cleanse your space—you can do this by burning sage or incense sticks. A good way to help cleanse rooms is to put a bowl of water in one corner of the room, a small bowl of salt in the second, a candle in the third corner and a burning incense stick in the fourth (obviously, you need to ensure that there is nothing flammable nearby); you can then open all the windows in the room to allow the old energy to disperse and bring in the new energies.

Once you have completed this, create a mandala of crystals in the room, or you could create an altar incorporating seasonal essential oils, such as frankincense, myrrh, nutmeg, or orange.

A fun present—especially at Christmas, when it is traditionally published—is a copy of *Old Moore's Almanac*—it has been published annually since 1697 and contains predictions based on astrology for the upcoming year.

QUESTIONS ON CHAPTER 9

1. Determine what your astrological moon sign is and analyze how it affects you when added to your sun sign.
2. List the planets and their corresponding crystals.
3. Suggest ways you can use astrology and crystals together.
4. Explain how you can work on your birth chart with crystals.

CHAPTER 10

USING CRYSTALS TO CONNECT WITH GUIDES, ANGELS, AND ASCENDED MASTERS

Crystals are amazing tools to help us to connect with and feel the energy of the angelic realms. Many people use crystals to help call in and connect with different spiritual frequencies—which can be angelic, ascended masters, or other spiritual entities that manifest as guides, such as Native American Indians—and in this chapter I will give you information on how to do this. You can create the link in several ways. In appendix 2 at the back of the book there are some suggested crystal grid placements for connecting with archangels. You can also use crystals placed on an altar you have created with a specific spiritual frequency in mind—for example, if you want to work with St. Germain, who represents the purple flame, you could cover the altar with some purple fabric and place a piece of amethyst on the altar. You could display his picture and burn a purple candle to help invoke his energy, perhaps alongside some purple flowers. Alternatively, you can simply program a crystal or piece of jewelry to invoke the energy of the angel or guide you wish to stay close to, which you can then wear or carry around with you.

ANGELS AND THE ANGELIC HIERARCHY

● ● ● ● ● ● ● ○ ○ ○ ● ● ● ● · · ● ● ● ●

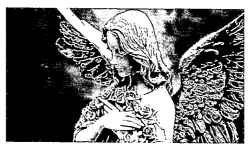

Traditional image of an angel

Many people find that their first esoteric encounters are with angels, and to some extent this is very apt as angels are perceived as messengers from God or the divine and so act as a bridge between heaven and earth. They have never incarnated within a physical body in the main, and are said to be androgynous. They only ever provide support to us as we travel through the earthly realm, with all its trials and tribulations.

The Bible tells us that angels were created by God in order to support creation as a whole, and therefore every plant, animal, planet, and even crystals are linked to angelic intelligence and presence. Interestingly, they are also mentioned in other religions and cultures, such as Islam, Buddhism, and Judaism. They are here to inspire and are often associated with beauty, love, peace, and harmony.

There are several different categories, or "spheres," of angels.

Sphere 1

Sphere 1 includes:

Seraphim

- Highest order of angels—closest to God/the creator
- Acknowledged in the Old Testament
- Work with sound to balance movement of planets, stars, and heavens.

Cherubim

- Guardians of light, holding and guarding the energy of the sun, moon, and stars.

Thrones

- Aligned to the presence of God
- Look after and guard the planets.

Sphere 2

This sphere includes:

Dominions

- Oversee lower-level angelic realms
- Help us to navigate the passage between spiritual and physical realms
- Depicted as carrying a golden staff in the right hand and a scepter or orb in the left.

Virtues

- Transmit beams of divine light
- Responsible for manifesting miracles.

Powers

- Keepers of the Akashic records (records of all thoughts/actions of each soul)
- Protect our souls and the world from evil
- Angels of birth and death.

Sphere 3

The third sphere includes:

Principalities

- Guardians of countries, towns, cities, villages, sacred sites
- Oversee the work of the angels below them
- Guides to religious leaders.

Archangels

- Most widely known; e.g., Michael, Gabriel, Raphael, Uriel

- Lead bands of angels and oversee their work
- Are omnipresent.

Angels

- Closest to humanity and have various responsibilities (e.g., angels of joy, peace, love, hope, healing). Guardian angels fall into this category.

ARCHANGELS

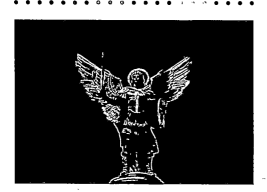

An archangel

The New Testament refers to seven archangels—Michael, Gabriel, Raphael, Uriel, Raguel, Seraphiel and Haniel. They are the chief angels and are the ones who bear divine decrees—such as Gabriel, who appeared when Jesus was born. Although there are said to be millions of archangels throughout the universe, the four most closely connected with earth are Michael, Raphael, Gabriel, and Uriel. Other archangels often referred to are Ariel, Azrael, Chamuel, Haniel, Jeremiel, Jophiel, Metatron, Raguel, Raziel, Sandalphon, and Zadkiel.

Although they are not ascribed a gender, a specific angelic energy can sometimes be discerned as masculine or feminine, and this is often linked to the role that the angel plays. Archangel Michael is often referred to as masculine, while Archangel Ariel is perceived as feminine.

The four main archangels

Archangel	Gabriel
Colour/Ray	White
Virtue	Purity

Archangel	Michael
Colour/Ray	Blue
Virtue	Will

Archangel	Raphael
Colour/Ray	Green
Virtue	Healing

Archangel	Uriel
Colour/Ray	Gold
Virtue	Peace

Entitled colors of the archangels. Different cultures hold different colors of significance for the archangels, so although the colors shown are commonly accepted and used there may be some variations according to source.

Archangel Michael

Michael is the head of all archangels. He offers protection (physical, emotional, and psychical), courage, strength, truth, and integrity. His chief function is to calm fear.

He is often seen with a sword, which he uses to protect us from negative energies. Colors associated with Michael are bright blue or purple light. Michael helps us to understand our life's purpose, so he offers help when our beliefs are challenged; when we lack motivation, direction, or vitality; if we suffer from low self-esteem; or are in need of courage. He should be invoked when you feel you need protection or wish to do space clearing. Specific crystals associated with Michael include amethyst, hematite, lapis lazuli, and smoky quartz.

Archangel Raphael

Raphael is the archangel who works with healers and assists with all forms of healing, including working with addictions. If called upon, he helps to rapidly heal body, mind, and spirit. His energy is loving, kind, and gentle, and the color green is associated with his energy. Raphael is also linked with animals and travel. Crystals associated with Raphael include malachite, chrysoprase, green calcite, emerald, and prehnite.

Archangel Gabriel

Sometimes depicted as female in art and literature, Gabriel is known as God's messenger. Gabriel and Michael are the only angels mentioned by name in the Old Testament. Archangel Gabriel will help those who need to make changes in their lives. This archangel can support all forms of communication and inspires artists, writers, etc. The color white is associated with his energy. Crystals aligned with Gabriel's energy include carnelian, celestite, citrine, and garnet.

Archangel Uriel

Uriel is associated with warnings of natural disasters, weather, and earth changes (Uriel warned Noah of the impending flood). He can offer healing in the aftermath of these occurrences and so is linked to earth healing. He is also linked to spiritual connection and alchemy. The color gold is associated with his energy. Crystals that may help to connect to Uriel include amethyst, labradorite, fluorite, and pyrite.

GUARDIAN ANGELS

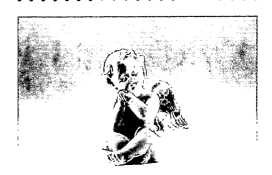

A cherub guardian angel

Most people understand the concept of a guardian angel. A guardian angel is assigned to every incarnated individual on the planet at birth, and the role of these angels is to guide and support us on our path as we grow and progress on earth. We need to invite angels into our lives as they can help only when we ask.

Guardian angels bring comfort and support during difficult and trying times. Their energies are most tangible in times when danger, grief, despair, or illness begin to engulf us. Conversely, they are also tangible when we encounter moments of intense joy, such as the birth of a child.

It is said that we incarnate with free will, and therefore angels must be called in by the individual, although others believe that the guardian angel is linked to our higher self—our soul essence, rather our physical, human self.

CONTACTING YOUR GUARDIAN ANGEL

Here is an exercise you can do to link with your guardian angel, and a meditation that you can do to help aid your connection.

Sit and try to empty your mind. If you have a meditation ritual, that is fine to use. Trust your intuition and awareness of things happening around you. When I first did this exercise many years ago, I was aware of something stroking my cheek. This happened every time I tried to link with my angels, and eventually I gave in and accepted that this was their way of contacting me. You can use crystals that are already predisposed to angel frequencies to help the process.

There is a list at the end of this chapter, but also be guided by your own intuition (and that of your guardian angel!).

You may also wish to light a candle and burn some essential oils or incense.

Imagine you are in a place where you are at your most relaxed—this could be walking in nature, lying on a beach, sitting in a cave, or anywhere else you can fully visualize yourself being. Try to conjure up the fragrances and sensations in your mind of where you are placing yourself. You don't have to "see," "hear," or "smell" them—just use your imagination to take yourself to that place you are creating in your mind.

Now, as you relax, begin to visualize a light in front of you—it may be white or have tinges of pastel colors within it. Just go with whatever your imagination is showing you. Move forward and step into the color, feel the color surround your aura.

Become aware of a passage of light that draws you forward into a room; the door is open, you feel a safe and loving energy connecting with you, and you perceive a sense of peace and tranquility, which starts to build within your being.

As this sense of peace and tranquility becomes stronger, be aware of a presence in the center and walk toward the presence—this is your guardian angel. Allow your guardian angel to walk into your energy field, and get a sense of how this connection feels.

Once you have made this connection you can ask your guardian angel's name; this may come as a color or an energy, and often when you connect with angelic frequencies the energy can feel cool or sparkly. Take this time to commune with your guardian angel and allow thoughts to merely drop into your consciousness if you can.

When the time is right, allow your guardian angel to step back—knowing that you can make this connection again at any time or place of your choice.

Bring your focus back into the room and become aware of your body on the floor or chair and your feet on the ground. Take two or three deep breaths, and, when you are ready, bring your focus fully back and open your eyes. You may wish to eat something sweet or drink some water as this will help to ground you.

Once you have completed the meditation above, try to open your awareness to things happening around you. Are you seeing a phrase or image being represented everywhere? Is there some music or a film that you are suddenly drawn to? Do you have instincts or thoughts that keep dropping into your mind? These are common ways that angels make their presence felt.

CRYSTALS WITH AN ANGELIC ENERGY AND ANGELIC "SIGNALS"

Crystals with an angelic energy

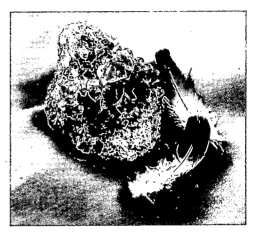

Tools to invoke angelic energies

Apophyllite
Selenite
Angelite
Golden rutilated quartz
Celestine
Angel aura
Prehnite
Amethyst

Angelic "signals"

Feathers: This is one of the most common ways of communication. The feathers appear in odd places. I once found a feather in my conservatory after I had just watched a TV interview about angels. Before the interview I had hoovered the conservatory and all the windows and doors were closed. I stopped the hoovering to watch the TV interview and when I returned to the conservatory there was a big white feather right in the middle of the floor!

Cloud formations: These often can be seen over sacred sites, but also if you are asking for guidance or evidence of angels' presence, you may see clouds form into angelic or feather shapes.

Words: Many people are familiar with angel cards, which contain only one word and, when the card is drawn from the pack, the word should have a significance for the person taking the card. This can be guidance for you, giving you an indication of what you need to be aware of to help support and steer you.

Crystals: When working with crystals—especially clear quartz—you can often "see" angels or feathers. This is called **scrying**, but it could indicate an angelic quality is held for you within that crystal.

Car parking: Many angelic enthusiasts report that they ask their angels to provide a car parking space for them! I've never been successful with this, but I think my concern is that my angel has more important things to do for me. However, I am working on my perception as I am sure that my angel will be more than happy to do this for me!

You have nothing to lose by testing out these theories . Ask your angel to confirm your mutual connection in the best way possible, and then sit back and wait for feathers, cloud formations, synchronicity, and so on, which will come to you in a short space of time. However, when your guardian angel has gone to all the trouble of contacting you, please don't dismiss it as a coincidence—be amazed and grateful: this will ensure a deeper and more tangible connection is forged.

INTERESTING INFORMATION

The four main archangels each have specific correspondences:

Archangel of the South: Call upon Archangel Michael when you feel you need help with physical matters, protection, trust, or vitality. Physical representations of Archangel Michael are the sun, essential oils, candles, and fire.

Archangel of the North: Archangel Uriel's responsibilities include science and technology, philosophy, wisdom, and transformation. Physical representations

of Archangel Uriel are crystals, religious or spiritual imagery, and the earth.

Archangel of the West: Archangel Gabriel's corresponding responsibilities are emotions, intuition, inspiration, and change. Physical representations of Archangel Gabriel are the moon, water, and mirrors.

Archangel of the East: Archangel Raphael represents enlightenment, creativity, and clarity. Physical representations of Archangel Raphael are incense, feathers, chiming bells, and air.

CONNECTING WITH SPIRIT GUIDES

Many spirit guides are Native American Indians

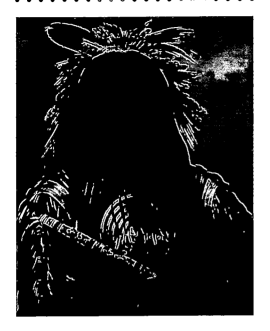

Many people believe that everyone has a group of spirit guides, which appear in different forms and with differing skills and purposes and who are there to support our spiritual growth and awareness, just as everyone has a guardian angel who is there to protect and care for our spiritual well-being.

Spirit guides can take many guises, which may be of someone who has lived and is now deceased—perhaps a relative—or of discarnate energies that appear as popular archetypes, such as Native American Indians or ancient Chinese seers or Australian Aborigines.

INTERESTING INFORMATION

Spirit guides are beings of light who support your incarnated soul (you) to reach your highest potential.

- Spirit guides are your direct link to the spirit world.
- Even though you may not be aware of it, your guides have always been alongside you, from the time of your conception. Some people believe that when young children have "invisible friends" they are in contact with their spirit guides. This contact diminishes as they become more embroiled in the material world; however, some lucky people never lose their connection and go on to develop naturally as mediums, clairvoyants, or healers, but we can all reconnect with a little patience and practice.

- You have multiple spirit guides in one lifetime; these different guides support different aspects of our lives and spiritual development by helping us to realize our purpose for incarnating on earth.
- Spirit guides are sent to guide us but not to control us—part of the "rules" when we incarnate is that we can exercise free will, so they cannot stop us from doing things even when it may not be for our greater good.
- Spirit guides are usually beings who possess levels of mastery in particular aspects of existence, which is what they are assigned to support us with.

Power animals

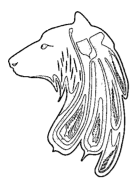

A power animal

Power animals are another form of guide and have their roots in shamanism (an ancient healing tradition which has roots in a number of indigenous cultures all over the world). Each power animal has an attribute; for example, deer are associated both with soft, gentle qualities and with strength and determination, while a butterfly totem or power animal communicates the ability to go through important changes with grace and lightness.

Other guides

Other more unusual connections with guides may be formed through the faerie or nature kingdoms—think of the leprechauns associated with Ireland and Cornwall—or even interdimensional beings from space.

Making the connection

People find that they can connect with their guides in a vast number of ways. A few examples are:

- **Via dream states**—sometimes you can remember a dream that gives you a solution to a problem, or you just wake up with knowledge that you didn't have before you went to sleep.
- **In meditation**—through visualization, bringing messages through thought processes or urges, which can provide insight or guidance.
- **A "shift" in your energy field**—sometimes perceived as a change of temperature (usually colder) or a deeper sense of peace and stillness.
- **A sudden strong sense**—which could be of peace or reassurance, decisiveness or simply peace. You might also feel a strong "gut" feeling about a situation or decision being right or wrong.
- **Via tarot cards, angel cards, angel boards, etc.**—or it might be something random like a magazine you have picked up in a waiting room that contains an article that provides you with information specific to you at that time.
- **External signs**—such as suddenly being aware of a billboard that has significance to you, or a piece of music being played on the radio that has words that resonate with you. Another sign can be flickering lights or sounds that come from nowhere.
- **Physical sensations**—can include your hair being ruffled or a hand placed on your body. This is often reported during reiki healing sessions, where recipients say that it sometimes feels as though two people are doing the treatment as they can feel two pairs of hands instead of one!

Connection with guides can feel like you are receiving wise, kind advice that will assist you in following your life's purpose, but also conveys a sense of unconditional love. Guides are there to ensure that we are guided and steered to make the right decisions to help us achieve the goals we are meant to reach in our current lifetime on earth. They are the reason for the synchronicity or coincidences that occur in our lives from time to time. When you are trying to connect and work with your angels you will find that their presence is stronger the more you relax and trust the connections you make.

ASCENDED MASTERS

The ascended masters are also known as the White Brotherhood. People who claim to have channeled them include Madame Blavatsky, Alice Bailey, Elizabeth Prophet, and Edmund Harrold.

Ascended masters are reputed to be souls who have ascended to a higher dimension of being because they have lived several incarnated lives that have served humanity well.

Different ascended masters have different attributes.

Kathumi

Attributes:
Relationships, connections
Animal kingdom, crystal and earth kingdom
Interconnection with all living things
St. Francis of Assisi
Vital life-force connection, ley lines,
    vortexes.

Suggested crystals: yellow calcite, black obsidian.

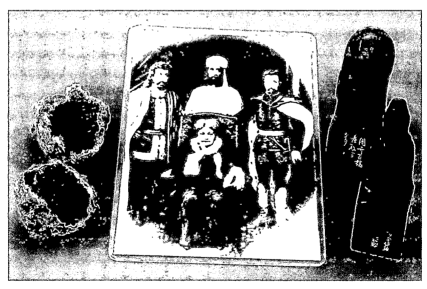

This is an image of Madame Blavatsky, who founded the Theosophical Society and is author of Isis Unveiled as well as other spiritual books. The picture is reputed to show her (in the middle) with three of her guides and teachers: from the left, Kathumi, El Morya, and St. Germain.

Mother Mary

Attributes:
Gentle energy
Madonna blue
Nurturing, divine mother energy
Loving all beings
Fed with knowledge, wisdom
Feminine power
Energy flow, connections with cycles,
    seasons, birth.

Suggested crystals: blue quartz, white
agate.

Lady Nada

Attributes:
Mary Magdalene, Jesus, and Mother Mary
    all soulmates
Solar feminine qualities
Joy, innocence, purity
Sensuality and sexuality
Springtime
Inner-child connection
Beginnings.

Suggested crystals: rose quartz,
apophyllite.

Jesus

Also known as Sananda.

Attributes:
Ray of manifestation
Conduit for Christ force—Matraiya energy
Ruby flame carried by Jesus

Loving passionate, gentle, intense passion
    for mankind, faith in us, very strong,
    clear, aligned
Truth, wisdom, physical anchoring
Expanding consciousness, opening the
    heart, finding the divinity.

Suggested crystals: garnet, pyrite.

Lady Portia

Attributes:
St. Germain's soul mate
Linked with Morgan Le Fay—they are
    believed to be the same ascended master
    who incarnated into two different
    lifetimes as these individual personalities
Keeper of the Sacred Heart Flame
Guardian of the way, challenger, can be dark
    and sinister but to achieve a positive end
Governs judgement and balance
Creator of harmony and also goddess of
    justice and karma release
Feminine power, focused on endings and
    beginnings
Color dark violet
Transformation through feminine ways
Magical and mystical
Atlantis
Black lady in Shakespeare's plays.

Suggested crystals: amethyst, clear quartz,
pyrite, and sodalite.

St. Germain

Was Francis Bacon, Merlin, Christopher
Columbus.

Attributes:
Teaches through challenge and the violet ray
    of alchemy
Custodian of the violet flame
Ceremony, ritual, magic
Wonder man of Europe
Advisor of Napoleon
Works with "I am" affirmations.

Suggested crystals: amethyst, fluorite.

El Moraya

Incarnated as King Arthur, El Moraya was
also an Indian prince.

Attributes:
Represents equilibrium, leadership, balance,
    strength
Strong blue color
Very matter of fact
Protector, powerful
Strategy, consciousness
Gentle, loyal, passionate, recognizing the
    existence of unconditional love
Master of discipline.

Suggested crystals: lapis lazuli, sodalite.

Kwan Yin

Attributes:
Worshipped as a goddess of compassion in
    China
Represents powers of compassion
Opalescent pearl
Order, compassion, discipline, powerful.

Suggested crystals: pearl, moonstone.

Dwal Khul

Attributes:
Chaos leading to order
Serene, smiling, quietly joyous, peaceful
Possession and demons
Youngest ascended master who wrote
    through Alice Bailey
Origins in Tibet.

Suggested crystals: carnelian, snowflake
obsidian.

Serapis Bay

Attributes:
Smell of the ocean, clear, pine
Atlantean, Egyptian
Angels incarnate on the planet
Bridge between masters and archangels
Grace and flow.

Suggested crystals: turquoise, labradorite.

CRYSTAL DIVINATION

Dowsing

A relatively simple way of divination is to
use a crystal pendulum to ask questions.
Some people keep a pendulum specifically
for this purpose. You can hold the pendulum
in the middle of the diagram shown. Once
you have asked the question, allow it to
swing in the direction of the correct answer.

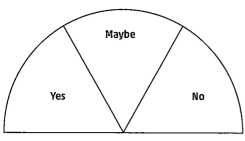

Dowsing chart. There is a larger version of this chart in appendix 6.

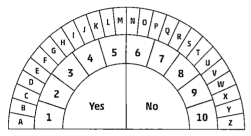

Dowsing number chart. There is a larger version of this chart in appendix 6.

Scrying, or crystallomancy

The standard picture of a psychic reading is that of a person sitting at a table holding a crystal ball. This practice is known as scrying, or crystallomancy, and has been around for hundreds of years. Queen Elizabeth I used to have readings by John Dee, who was one of her advisors, and his tools are still on display at the British Museum. Quartz crystal isn't the only stone that can be used for scrying—sometimes available are black obsidian discs, which can be used to discern reflections within them—a bit like a mirror.

Using a crystal ball to give a scrying reading

When you purchase a crystal ball for this purpose it is best to select one that has lots of inclusions and rainbows within it rather than one that is perfectly clear. Many readers cover their crystal spheres in silk when they are not in use, to keep them clear of any other energies, but usually prior to starting a reading will perform a cleansing ritual upon the crystal ball and themselves, as well as ensuring that they are grounded and centered.

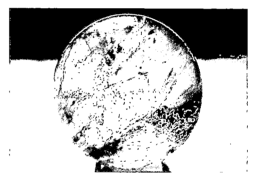

Crystal ball

It is not a process that you can rush. Here are some steps to help you achieve a successful reading, but remember that it takes time, patience, and practice to master this skill.

• If you are doing the reading for yourself it may help to focus on what you want answers for—if you are doing the reading for someone else, you may or may not wish to ask questions.

- Light a candle and perhaps burn some incense or essential oils. Ensure that phones are turned off so that you aren't interrupted.
- Many people choose to hold the crystal ball in their hands, while others hold it within a silk scarf.
- Take two or three deep breaths and let your eyes go in and out of focus. (This can be similar to when you gaze at a flickering candle and you can see the "aura" around the flame.)
- You may see images or symbols that appear within the crystal sphere. Try to interpret the significance of these pictures, either for yourself or the person receiving the reading. If you are struggling with the interpretation you can write them down and revisit them another day.

Lithomancy—casting stones

The stones that you use for lithomancy could be runes, or you could use a set of tumble stones. The advantage of using runes is that the symbols carved into the stones each have a significant meaning, which can help with adding more depth to a reading. However, you could create a set of stones that are specific to you, or link to sacred geometry or astrology (planets and houses), for example. If you choose to keep it simple and just have tumble stones, ensure that you select a set that are not similar in correspondences and color. To take care of your crystals, you should try to ensure that they are similar in hardness so that they don't scratch one another. For this reason, any crystals from the quartz family would

be a good selection, such as amethyst, rose quartz, citrine, aventurine, and carnelian.

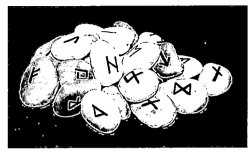
Crystal rune stones

There are several ways that you can use your casting stones. Here are a couple of ideas (but always remember to cleanse your crystals before and after use):

- You could simply place them in a bag and choose three stones by taking them out of the bag without looking at what you are picking. The significance of the stones you choose could be akin to a three-card tarot spread, with the first crystal chosen having significance for past influences, the second present, and the third future. If you are skilled at attuning to crystals, you will find that you can work creatively with them in this way. If you are less confidence with attuning, you can go by standard crystal correspondences, but it probably won't have the same depth of message—what an incentive to keep practicing your attunement abilities!
- You can make your own casting boards. The one illustrated uses a template for an astrological chart, but you could make one as simple or as complicated as you wish. Then select about five or six stones from the bag without

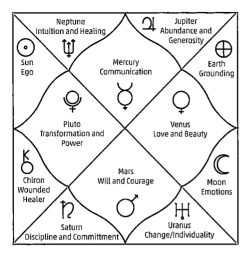 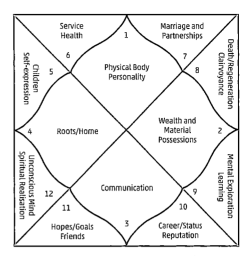

Crystal casting boards. There are larger versions of these and more information in appendix 5.

looking at what you are taking. Hold all the stones in between the palms of your hands and take a moment to ground and center yourself and ask any questions that you wish to have answers to. With your hands about two to three inches(5–7.5 cm) above the casting board, allow the stones to drop onto the board. The spaces the crystals land upon will have a significance, and then it is just a question of interpreting the reading by linking the significance of where they have landed to the properties of each crystal.

QUESTIONS ON CHAPTER 10

1. Name the four archangels and their correspondences.
2. Suggest four crystals that could help you connect with angels.
3. What is the difference between a guide and a power animal?
4. Explain who the ascended masters are.
5. What is the difference between scrying with a crystal and lithomancy?

CHAPTER 11

● ● ○ ● (●

SPACE CLEARING WITH CRYSTALS

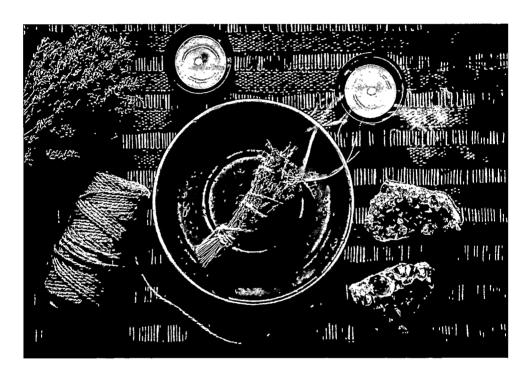

Nowadays more and more people are spending a greater amount of time in their homes. Only a few years ago it was the place we could retreat to from the hustle and bustle of the world. However, these days many of us are expected to work from home, which can create all sorts of energy dynamics. This can be exacerbated when two or more people are trying to work from the same place, with perhaps some home schooling thrown in. This may mean that your home no longer has the recharging and realigning atmosphere that it once did. The increased electromagnetic frequency use, the stress levels previously contained to some extent at the office, lack of privacy, and possibly constant interruptions when trying to focus, etc., can impact on the energy of your home, making it difficult to feel that it is the place of sanctity and protection it once was.

WAYS YOU CAN USE CRYSTALS FOR SPACE CLEARING

First of all, let's break down the different types of energy clearance you might need to create. I would say that they fall into three main categories:

• Electromagnetic-field energy
• Geopathic energy
• Energy in a specific room.

Electromagnetic-field (EMF) energy clearance

EMFs come from power inlets into your house; electrical devices you use such as Wi-Fi networks; and household appliances like smart meters, microwaves, computers, fluorescent lighting, cordless/cell phones, etc.; as well as outside sources from electricity pylons, television masts, cell-phone masts, and so on. Even your Fitbit is generating EMF pollution, so wearing it 24/7 might not be the healthiest thing for you. Our lives are awash with electromagnetic pollution, both inside and outside the home, so it makes sense to try to minimize it in your home—particularly the bedroom area where you sleep—as much as possible.

You can buy an EMF meter to measure the pollution emitted. When using crystals to clear the energy, the meter can show you the difference before and after you have placed your chosen crystals to counteract the EMF. However, some of you more sensitive souls out there will probably be able to sense the difference in the energy. Some people find that with a reduction in EMF they no longer suffer from common complaints such as headaches, allergies, tiredness, insomnia, and a host of other symptoms of EMF hypersensitivity. With the advent of 5G this may well be something that will continue to grow in both awareness and concern for the health issues it can create.

Geopathic energy clearance

Geopathic energy is stagnant energy that comes from the earth, buildings, or roads that have been inappropriately placed in the landscape. There can be many reasons this negative energy is generated:

• Energy vortexes can be created by water underneath a property (for example, a disused well) or by the memory of trauma that can be left following disturbing or traumatic events occurring on or in a property.
• Ley lines are energy lines that flow along the earth (known as fairy paths to the Irish, dragon lines to the Chinese, and spirit lines by the Peruvians). Wikipedia defines them as "intentionally straight alignments drawn between various historic structures and prominent landmarks."[1] Their existence was suggested in 1921 by Alfred Watkins, whose book *The Old Straight Track*[2] shared his thoughts that this is how homing animals like pigeons find their

---

[1]Wikipedia contributors, "Ley Line," *Wikipedia, the Free Encyclopedia*, https://en.wikipedia.org/w/index.php?title=Ley_line&oldid=1057215123 (accessed November 30, 2021).
[2]Head of Zeus, 2014.

RECOMMENDED CRYSTALS

Along with some of the facts given here, the power of your intention will intensify the action of the crystal, so programming a crystal to protect against negative energies will further empower the work that it does.

- **Shungite:** All over the internet you will see that shungite is the "go-to" crystal for EMF reduction. It has absorbing and shielding properties that are scientifically proven. In industry, shungite is used in a variety of ways, such as in paint, concrete, and particle boards to aid protection against EMF. Considered to be the miracle stone of the twenty-first century, shungite is mined in Karelia in Russia. Black in color, shungite is up to 98% carbon and contains something called fullerene carbon (Buckminsterfullerene is a type of fullerene and was discovered by Richard Smalley, Robert Curl, and Harry Kroto in 1985. They were awarded the Nobel Prize in 1996 for this discovery). Fullerenes have many scientific applications: in solar cells, antiviral agents, and antioxidants, to name a few. As well as carbon, a variety of other elements may be present in shungite.

- **Amethyst:** I personally have used amethyst to help clear the EMF in a small farm that was surrounded by electricity pylons. A master dowser had checked the site and had attempted to clear it, but was struggling to get a reading that indicated that the energy was entirely clear. We planted several small pieces of amethyst druse in the ground and, according to the master dowser, that finally cleared the energy generated by the pylons.

- **Rose quartz:** This contains titanium, which is used to make containers for nuclear waste. Perhaps this is the reason it seems to work well when used to help disperse EMF.

- **Black tourmaline:** This is a tried-and-tested, heavy-duty protection stone. When you are using black tourmaline ensure that you cleanse it regularly, as it tends to have an absorbing energy rather than a blocking energy, so in effect it will hold energy rather than disperse it.

way back to their nests. If a house is sitting on crossed ley lines, this can influence the energy of the house. Rose quartz is often the stone of choice for these types of energies, although selenite and of course black tourmaline are also recommended. If you can locate the specific place where, for example, an energy vortex occurs—and this is usually done by dowsing—you can simply place the crystal on that location to minimize the negative energy. If you want to find out more about how this is done, contact the American Society of Dowsers or the

British Society of Dowsers, who have a lot of information and offer training and workshops and will be able to recommend expert dowsers to you.

Crystals to protect and enhance the energy in specific rooms

Elsewhere in this book you will find recommendations for crystals, such as carnelian, apophyllite, and black tourmaline, that identify different levels of personal protection that might be required.

In cases of serious negative energy, I would always recommend black tourmaline—this can be placed in specific rooms, or you can place it by the entrance to your home. Alternatively, you could "grid" the house by placing a piece in each corner of the property, either inside it or outside—if you have a back yard, place it there. With crystals the power of your intention is important, so I would recommend programming them with specific instructions, such as "protect this home and all who live here," along with regular cleansing of the crystals.

It should be said that loving energies can help to neutralize and purify stagnant and negative energies, as well as using rose quartz, particularly in rooms where there have been arguments. Clarifying crystals, such as clear quartz or an amethyst geode, will have a positive effect on all who are around them.

In other rooms, such as a study or workroom, you might want to stimulate

creativity and communication, so using blue crystals like sodalite or blue quartz or energizing crystals like citrine and carnelian would help, especially if placed on your desk, for example.

Another way of energizing a room is to have a pretty bowl containing water in the room. You can place crystals into the water and add Bach flower remedies, or other gem or flower remedies that have a cleansing and clearing quality. Adding flowers or flower petals really makes the bowl a feature. I often use this as a centerpiece when I have people to dinner. Alternatively, you can make a "crystal garden," again using an attractive container, which you fill with decorative sand (this can be bought from aquatic stores). Arrange some crystals of your choice on the sand—you could also place an incense burner in the arrangement.

Other space-clearing tools you can use include crystal bowls; incense works very well, as well as Palo Santo, a sacred wood that when burned gives off a lovely smell, which immediately lifts the energy of a room or group of people.

Creating custom-made crystal grids will work well when you have a specific focus. You may choose to place a grid around your bed to ensure a good night's sleep, for example. Using a grid in a room that has many uses or is used by lots of different people helps to set the energy (for example, if you work in a therapy center that rents out the room to other people). Bringing some crystals with you every time you are there will calibrate the energy to a frequency that is best for you and your clients.

I have known people who are having extensions built to place rose quartz into the foundations. Remember—if you use directional crystals (crystals with a point), by pointing them inward you will draw energy into the building/room, and by placing them pointing outward you will be dispersing energy away.

QUESTIONS ON CHAPTER 11

1. Try different types of crystals that are protective and decide which one is for you. Deeply protective black tourmaline might be keeping friends and family at bay but could make you seem a little cut off from them; apophyllite could make you feel ungrounded and a bit spacy. But everyone is different—work out which crystal works best for you and buy some jewelry so that you can wear your protection as unobtrusively as possible.

2. Try cleansing a room on a regular basis where there can sometimes be stress—for example, your home office, or perhaps the kitchen. Be mindful of the changes in the energies of the room when you have cleansed compared with when you haven't. We spend a lot of time in our kitchens, and every evening I light a candle to bring in light to that particular room.

● ● ○ ● ◌ ●

CHAPTER 12

NUMEROLOGY

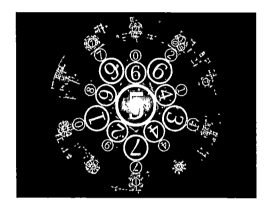

In the same way that our star sign is said to represent our personalities and talents, numerologists consider that numbers, calculated by adding together your date-of-birth numbers, can help you ascertain what your life path and gifts are.

Below are some brief descriptions of the divine aspects of the numbers themselves.

NUMBER DEFINITIONS

● ● ● ● ● ● ● ○ ○ ○ ● ● ● ⌐ ⌐ ⌐ ● ● ● ●

0. Endings and beginnings, infinity—zero is not a life-path or destiny number, for it is not possible to calculate the numbers in numerology to zero

1. New beginnings, change, strength, leadership, innovation
2. Balance, harmony, resilience, peacemaking, cooperation
3. Communication/interaction, creation, inspiration
4. Organization, planning, design, efficiency, integrity
5. Action, restlessness, adventure, freedom, pushing boundaries
6. Nurturing, responsibility
7. Consciousness, truth seeking, spiritual path
8. Power, taking charge, entrepreneurialism
9. Humanitarianism, improving humanity, and making the world a better place
10. Rebirth.

DIGIT SUMMING

● ● ● ● ● ● ● ● ○ ○ ○ ● ● ● ○ ○ ⌐ ● ● ●

Numerologists reduce a number or word by a process known as digit summing. The energy conclusion is based on the single digit that is produced. This involves taking the sum of all the digits in a number (or the digits that the letters in a word correspond to) and repeating the process until a single-digit answer is produced. See table below for the numbers assigned to each letter.

1	2	3	4	5	6	7	8	9
A	B	C	D	E	F	G	H	I
J	K	L	M	N	O	P	Q	R
S	T	U	V	W	X	Y	Z	

LIFE-PATH NUMBER

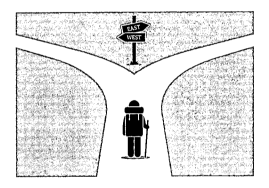

This number indicates the influences at play throughout your life. It is obtained by calculating your birth date and is similar to the sun sign in astrology, which is an indicator of your personality type, etc. It can show you positive and negative aspects, as does the sun sign in astrology, but remember that we have free will, so how we choose to navigate the highs and lows that we experience through life is down to our own responses. It can give insight, which we can use to inform and guide us if we wish.

Example:
John Fitzgerald Kennedy—date of birth: 29 May 1917

Step 1. Reduce the day.

2 + 9 = 11 (This is a master number (see explanation below) so we don't reduce it any further.)

Step 2. Reduce the month.

= 5 (There is only one digit, so it remains as 5.)

Step 3. Reduce the year.

1 + 9 + 1 + 7 = 18 (This is not a master number, so we reduce it further.)

1 + 8 = 9

Step 4. Reduce the three total numbers added together.

11 + 5 + 9 = 25 (This is not a master number, so we reduce it further.)

2 + 5 = 7

Life-path number: 7

DESTINY NUMBER

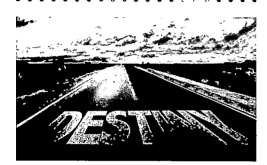

The destiny number is also known as the expression number. To calculate this, you use the letters of the names you were given at birth (including middle names—most people use the official name as it appears on your birth certificate). If you are known as Andy but your name is listed as Andrew, you would calculate your destiny number using Andrew rather than Andy. Once you've got the correct names you add the individual letter numbers together and reduce to a single digit, or master number. Each letter in your name corresponds to a number (see table above in "Digit Summing").

Example: Barry Roy Tappin

21997-967-217795

Now add each number in the sequence above together, as below:

Barry—2 + 1 + 9 + 9 + 7 = 28 (2 + 8 =10, 1 + 0 = 1)

The destiny number for Barry is 1.

Roy—9 + 6 + 7 = 22 (2 + 2 = 4)

The destiny number for Roy is 4.

Tappin—2 + 1 + 7 + 7 + 9 + 5 = 31 (3 + 1 = 4)

The destiny number for Tappin is 4.

Now you add all the destiny numbers together—in this case, 1 + 4 + 4 = 9. The final number is the destiny number—in this case, 9 for Barry Roy Tappin.

Your birth name is said to carry the energy of your current soul journey.

Example: John Fitzgerald Kennedy

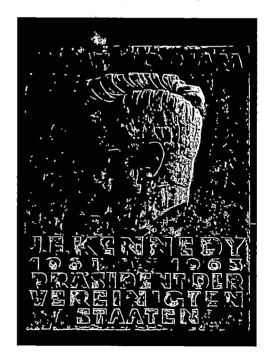

$$1 + 6 + 8 + 5 + 6 + 9 + 2 + 8 + 7 + 5 + 9 + 1 + 3 + 4 + 2 + 5 + 5 + 5 + 5 + 4 + 7 = 107$$

$$7 + 0 + 1 = 8$$

I will leave it to you to draw your own conclusions from the life-path and destiny numbers for President Kennedy given in the examples here. Perhaps you can try numerology out on other famous people to see what the numbers indicate for them.

MASTER NUMBERS

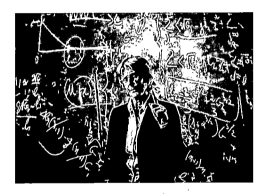

Some numbers carry more power in numerology than others. These are called master numbers. Although the single digits (1–9) are the most used in numerology, there are three double-digit numbers that indicate something more powerful. These are 11, 22, and 33 and are particularly relevant when calculating life-path or destiny numbers as above. Their correspondences are:

11. Cooperator, creator, and visualizer. Those who have 11 in their life-path or birth numbers tend to be empathic, spiritual, and intuitive.

22. Designer, builder. Again, anyone with 22 as a master number has a strong intuitive streak, but this is coupled with rational thought processes and the ability to actualize something of value and/or great meaning.

33. Deliverer, manifester. Sometimes known as the master or teacher, those with 33 can sometimes endure a difficult life, overcoming obstacles but also learning how to guide and heal others.

Often, these numbers become more important in later life as we start to realize and achieve our life purpose.

Below is a list of crystals whose energy supports the growth and learning that each number brings to an individual.

1. Sunstone
2. Sodalite
3. Carnelian
4. Hematite
5. Malachite
6. Moonstone
7. Amethyst
8. Citrine
9. Rose quartz

Master numbers

11. Selenite
22. Pyrite
33. Celestite

Finally, numerology can be used with crystals. Melody, in her book *Love Is in the Earth*,[1] calculated the numerology number

---

[1]Earth-Love Publishing, 1995.

of each crystal, making these crystals act as "touchstones" for people as they journey through life—a little like birthstones do in astrology. In this aspect, Melody has calculated the name by ascribing numbers to each letter of the crystal name.

Here are a few common examples from her book:

Life Path Number	Crystals
1	Angelite, aquamarine
2	Bismuth, shell
3	Lapis, amethyst
4	Clear quartz, apophyllite
5	Blue lace agate, amazonite
6	Jasper, green tourmaline
7	Agate, tiger iron
8	Jet, calcite
9	Malachite, unakite
11	Jade
22	Coral, galena
33	Ulexite, diamond

QUESTIONS ON CHAPTER 12

1. Why not try working out life-path numbers for well-known celebrities or close friends and family? Sometimes someone else's life-path number is easier to interpret than your own. Alternatively, ask friends and family how accurate they feel your life-path number is.

2. Think about or meditate on how you resonate with the crystals that link to your life-path number.

● ● ○ ● ◐ ●

CHAPTER 13

ANCESTRAL HEALING

WHAT IS ANCESTRAL HEALING?

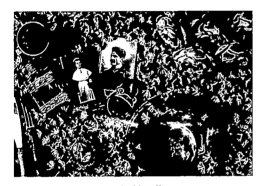

Ancestral healing

We all have an ancestral line that has had an influence on making us who we are. It has affected our DNA, our beliefs, our responses to various situations, our relationships, and our personality. The influence may have begun decades or even centuries ago, but the effects—both good and bad—continue to be passed through the family line. Ancestral healing is about releasing patterns, beliefs, and perhaps even ancestors who have influence over our lives today. On a personal level, it may allow us to get to the roots of a particular problem, but we can also help to heal the earth by healing negative occurrences such as wars, diseases, and other traumatic events.

Historically, many cultures have honored—and still do—their ancestors. These cultures can be found across the world, and include Native American Indians; Asian cultures in Cambodia, China, Japan, India, Thailand, Sri Lanka, Vietnam, the Philippines, and Indonesia; African cultures in ancient Egypt, Madagascar, Senegal, and Gambia; and in Europe the Celts and Romans.

These cultures acknowledge that although the ancestor is no longer incarnate on the planet there is still a connection between us. In our society we often explore this link via mediumship/spiritualism, and paganism and shamanism also work with ancestral connections to facilitate understanding and healing.

REASONS WHY ANCESTRAL HEALING IS REQUIRED

- **Trauma at the point of death:** this can include traumatic or unjust deaths, violent murders, etc., where the soul can become earthbound rather than passing into spirit in the normal way
- **Addictions,** such as alcoholism, that are passed down the family line

- **Health issues** passed down the family line
- **Dysfunctional relationships** with close family members; family archetypes such as dominating parents, siblings, etc.
- **Overattachment** to loved ones; **events that coincide with prior family events,** such as a child being born on the anniversary of a family member's death
- **Family curses:** well-known examples are the Guinness family and the Kennedy family, whose checkered family histories include tragedies that have befallen many family members over several generations
- **Family secrets:** although not always the case, family "sins" such as incest may be repeated by different family members, and other burdens of guilt and shame can pass down the family line, such as rejection, abandonment, betrayal, etc.

On a positive note, the reverse can also be true of working with ancestors. We may wish to maintain connections so that we can continue to receive the love and support we had from family members.

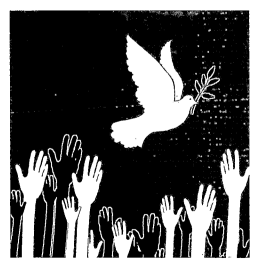
Dove

WAYS IN WHICH ANCESTRAL HEALING CAN BE DONE

Firstly, bear in mind that not everything is the fault of your ancestors. Everyone has their own karmic journey that is separate from family ties—a good astrologer can often identify this for you.

In order to release ancestral healing, you need to accept that you should be willing to forgive, and there are three aspects to this:

1. Acknowledge your pain/anger/resentment.
2. Ask for forgiveness from anyone you have hurt or harmed in this lifetime.
3. You need to be able to forgive yourself—there could be a reflection of aspects of yourself that requires acknowledgement too.

Many believe that there is a crystalline grid over the planet that holds the akashic records of humanity. Our energy system also retains a crystalline sheath, which holds our personal akashic records. Healing with crystals can help to clear the trauma or blocked energies of both the planet and ourselves. Techniques include:

- Guided visualization
- Communicating with/honoring the ancestors—some cultures have family altars, for example
- Spirit release—when the soul of the ancestor hasn't crossed over to the other side
- Various shamanic practices: drumming, journeying, etc.
- Crystal healing
- Cord cutting.

An attachment is a cord of energy that connects us to another person, like a telephone wire. These attachments can be positive and based on love, but more often they become an issue when we are connected because of anger, fear, or other unresolved issues, with either the living or those who have passed on. Phyllis Krystal is author of *Cutting the Ties That Bind*, in which she explores a wide range of cord-cutting techniques. When teaching students, I usually get them to visualize a figure of eight (crystals that are double terminated can be useful in this exercise) and to imagine themselves in one circle and the person, emotion, or situation that they wish to clear in the other. I ask them to feel the connection but then ask guides or angels, or alternatively visualize cutting between the two circles in any way that seems appropriate to them—this could be scissors, a knife, an axe, etc. Then, as the two circles disengage, they can send love or like to the other circle and healing to both themselves and the other person, situation, etc. Finally, it is probably best for them to then put some form of protection in place so that reconnection doesn't occur.

LETTING GO

1. Begin by bringing the person into your awareness and either picturing them or, ideally, having a photo of them near you.
2. Imagine a cord between the two of you that you are going to break, cut, or gently disengage from.
3. Try to identify the reason(s) for the release of the connection between you. This will empower the process and ensure that there is less likelihood of reconnection occurring through repetition of previous behavior, beliefs, etc.
4. Break/cut the cord, and send it back to the person with love. It may help to visualize them stepping back, being guided by spirit helpers or angels, etc., further into the light.
5. Return your energy to yourself and, where you felt the connection disengage, send healing or use a crystal such as selenite, clear quartz, or whatever you feel drawn to in order to protect and heal the area.

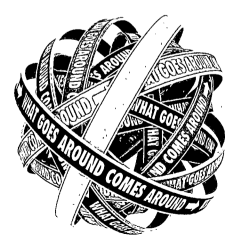

What goes around

Often, people will visit a medium to communicate with relatives who have passed on. I would recommend that you do research and ask for recommendations regarding mediums. The best place to go to may be your local spiritualist church. The National Spiritualist Association of Churches is one of the oldest and largest spiritualist church organizations in the United States, and can recommend genuine mediums. The Spiritualists' National Union in the UK has a code of conduct for all practicing mediums, and most spiritual churches in the UK belong to the SNU.

Regarding spirit release, this is best carried out with someone who has been trained to do it. The process can be extremely difficult or very easy, but I always refer students or clients on to specialist trained therapists or organizations such as the Spirit Release Foundation in the UK, which offers intensive training in this area and can advise and recommend healers who are competent in this work. Alternatively, Christian churches acknowledge this work too, and some priests and vicars are trained in exorcism, for example.

On a positive note, we are also able to continue to receive and tap into the energy, character, and skills of our ancestors, as well as receive the love and support we were able to enjoy while they were alive. Astrology provides us with insight as to the gifts, karma, challenges, and experiences an individual will encounter on their life journey, so we need to bear in mind that not everything is the fault of your ancestors— you have your own path to tread and experiences to encounter.

QUESTIONS ON CHAPTER 13

1. Ask around your family for copies of old photographs of ancestors—especially ones you didn't know—and try attuning to their photographs to get a feel for the energy of each person. Afterward you could discuss with other members of your family whether they have old stories about the people in the photographs or information on the work they did or type of person they were.
2. Try sending healing to your family line, which you can do in much the same way as you send distant or absent healing.

CHAPTER 14

● ● ○ ● ᛁ ●

COMBINING CRYSTALS WITH OTHER TREATMENTS

Hering's law of cure states that all healing starts from the head and moves down, from the inside out, and in reverse order as the symptoms have been acquired. Although Hering was a homeopath, this is a standard of philosophy that can be used by all holistic therapists. It indicates the direction of cure—that the healing process starts inside the body, and so often will not be directly evident. The symptoms on the outside of the body, the visible symptoms, are often the last to disappear. We should remember this when we are treating our clients and see no immediate effect. The initial changes in health are internal and imperceptible as we rebalance the life force and endeavor to return the body to homeostasis. The client will initially feel the changes mentally and emotionally. With continued treatment these changes will manifest in the physical and there can then be a visible change.

It is advisable to inform your client about treatment aftercare, perhaps in an aftercare leaflet. This should recommend that the client drink plenty of water for twenty-four hours after treatment, thus helping the body to eliminate toxins that have surfaced as a result of the treatment. It should

also include information on the healing crisis, and that it is not always a negative experience. It is important that the client is able to recognize symptoms of a healing crisis so that he or she does not become overly anxious. The client should be advised to try to relax as much as possible during this time. Hopefully when the crisis passes, the benefit of the treatment will be felt.

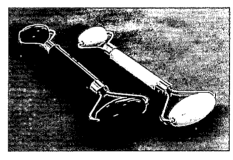

Crystal rollers

Crystal massage stones

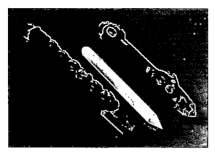

Crystal wands

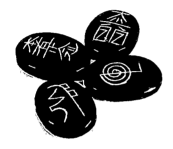

Crystals with reiki symbols

HOW TO COMBINE CRYSTALS WITH REFLEXOLOGY, REIKI, ACUPUNCTURE, AND MASSAGE

Adding crystals to almost any other therapy or treatment can enhance and customize the experience for the person receiving the treatment as well as the practitioner.

The following is by no means a definitive list of therapies that can incorporate crystals, but is intended to inspire everyone to consider the possibility of harnessing the energetic qualities of crystals to further empower other therapies.

Reflexology

Reflexology works on the principle that there are specific points in the hands and feet that connect to each organ in the body. Reflexologists believe that by applying pressure or stimulation on these points you can increase blood supply to an organ, thus improving circulation and releasing toxins. The treatment is usually very relaxing and can help the body to rebalance the circulatory system and also the life-force energy within the body, which in turn can support the body systems. Crystal wands or points can be used to stimulate the zones on the feet or hands. Instead of moving the crystal it should be held on a zone for around thirty seconds to two minutes. Using grounding crystals such as jasper or hematite on the foot chakra at the end of a treatment will help to ground a client. It is a gentle, safe, and relaxing treatment.

Massage

Stones can be placed under the couch where the massage will take place to create an ambient energy—see our crystal color baths in appendix 2 at the end of the book. Stones can also be used to massage a client in an area where, for example, muscles are tight. A simple chakra layout can be used and always works well. Hot-stone massage is a form of crystal healing, since the stones commonly used in this treatment are made of basalt, which is crystalline. Gem essences could also be incorporated into the massage blend.

Acupuncture

I have worked with some acupuncturists who have found that placing a crystal on a specific acupuncture point has significantly impacted on pulse readings.

Reiki

As with the massage treatments, you can incorporate a crystal grid—there are examples in appendix 2—to empower a reiki treatment. However, you could also program a crystal with the reiki symbols—here are just two examples:

- Having used a power symbol to program a crystal, you can give the crystal to your friend/client to take away and carry around, so that even if he or she is not attuned to reiki, the energy for continued healing effect can still be accessed.
- Using the distance-healing symbol, you could program a crystal with the intention that it sends energy to all the people you offer absent healing to. Some people write names in a book, while others place names in a healing basket. The programmed crystal can be placed on or alongside these to generate healing to all those requesting it.

SELECTING CRYSTALS FOR USE WITH OTHER THERAPIES

By selecting a crystal with properties that best suit the needs of the client/recipient, we can tailor a treatment to include balancing and enhancement of the subtle energy system (chakras, meridians, etc.). Selecting the correct crystals for everyone who is receiving the treatment is important, and often with beginners I suggest sticking to the "Fab 4" crystals—namely:

- Rose quartz—a crystal that promotes gentle unconditional love
- Clear quartz—which promotes clarity, purity, and energy detoxing
- Amethyst—which is healing, calming, and spiritual
- Hematite—which is grounding and gently protective.

WHY USE CRYSTALS?

- Rebalances the subtle energy system quickly and effectively
- Clients report a much deeper sense of relaxation and rejuvenation
- "Energy-aware" clients will report a sense of energy moving, thus deriving more from the treatment than merely a physical benefit
- Further enhancement of ALL holistic treatments.

OPTIONS WHEN USING CRYSTALS

- Dowsing chakras
- Energizing products used within the treatment
- Stimulating subtle energy points—chakras, meridians, marma points.
- Crystal "massage"
- Crystal layout
- Gem essences can be added to cleansing products, face masks, and massage mixes, but if the practitioner is qualified can also be applied to marma points, pressure points, and chakras.

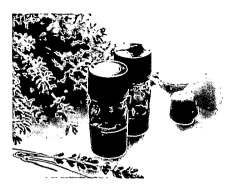

Gem essences

FACIAL MASSAGE

For the recipient, the massage combines the therapeutic physical benefits of a facial, including products and techniques, with the added healing energies of crystals, creating a truly holistic treatment benefiting mind, body, and spirit.

Massage is considered one of the oldest forms of healing. Regular facial massage can lead to smoother, firmer, more radiant skin by minimizing sagging and fine lines, releasing toxins and impurities, normalizing moisture balance, and releasing tension.

Crystals have a unique energy that resonates with the energies of our own body. By using crystals in the massage, they penetrate the energy systems of the whole body, clearing blockages in the energy system and rebalancing to make the person feel whole and relaxed.

Contraindications for facial massage

In certain situations, you should not carry out a facial massage on a client. The contraindications are as follows:

- High temperature or fever
- Acute infectious disease
- Skin or scalp infections
- Recent hemorrhage in treatment area
- Arthritis or osteoporosis in treatment area
- Any condition involving abnormally high muscle tone; e.g., spasticity, cerebral palsy, high muscle tone following head injury, stroke, etc.
- Recent head or neck injury
- Recent surgery
- Severe circulatory disorder
- Heart condition
- Thrombosis/embolism
- High or low blood pressure
- Dysfunction of the nervous system
- Epilepsy—due to the piezoelectrical charges from crystals it is advised that crystal therapists avoid the head area when working with someone who is epileptic
- Diabetes
- Any potentially fatal/terminal condition
- Recent scar tissue
- Severe bruising, open cuts, or abrasions
- Undiagnosed lumps, bumps, or swellings
- Allergies
- Migraine or headaches
- Mental ill health—some conditions may render crystal therapy non-therapeutic
- Pacemakers—due to the piezoelectrical charge in crystals it is recommended that additional care be taken with someone who has had a pacemaker fitted.

Equipment required

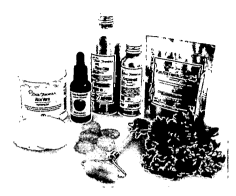

Materials for facial massage

1 bottle of cleanser
1 bottle of toner
1 bottle of oil
1 bottle of moisturizer
Mask ingredients
Gem essence
Cotton-wool pads
6 red jasper crystals—or other grounding
    crystals of your choice
6 rose quartz crystals—or other crystals of
    your choice
Massage stone of your choice
You will need a chair or couch to do this
    procedure.

Getting started

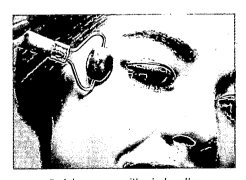

Facial massage with a jade roller

Before starting the treatment, make sure all jewelry or other objects are removed from yourself and the person you are working on so no injuries occur. Place the person on a chair that reclines slightly, or use a couch. To help the person relax, explain the procedure, then put some music on in the background and ask the person to close his or her eyes.

Ensure your hands are clean by washing them in soapy water or use a bactericidal hand cleanser before starting the procedure.

Set the scene

In an oil burner, with about a tablespoon of water or rose water, burn two or three drops of myrrh, neroli, and sandalwood essential oils. Alternatively, you can make a room spray with this recipe:

15 drops of myrrh
10 drops of neroli
15 drops of sandalwood
100 ml of chamomile flower water—
    sometimes known as hydrolat.

You can also add two to five drops of gem essence to either the oil burner or the spray if you wish.

The emotional freedom technique

The emotional freedom technique (EFT), just like acupuncture, works directly on the meridian system of the body. However, instead of using needles, during an EFT treatment the major meridian points are stimulated by tapping on them or massaging them lightly.

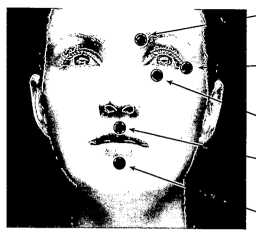

Relieves trauma and fear, aids energy levels, allows free expression and short-term memory recall

Relieves lethargy, increases energy levels, reinforces determination, gives clarity of thought, enables decision-making

Clears negative thought patterns and addictive or anxious behaviour, grounding

Clears feelings of panic, embarrassment and shock; relieves hunger pangs, and is also used to treat allergies

Stimulates chi flow, dissolves panic, anxiety and shame and removes fatigue

End points of the meridians used for the emotional freedom technique

Place a clear quartz point or tumble stone on these EFT points (shown in the figure), while asking the client to breathe in through the nose and out through the mouth at each point.

Face mask

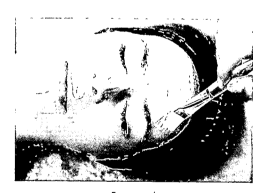

Face mask

Different face masks are available for different skin types, or you can make your own from natural ingredients such as:

- French green clay (good for oily skin)—contains minerals that the skin can absorb, such as magnesium, potassium, silica, calcium, selenium
- China/white clay (good for sensitive, dry skin)—contains zinc, silica, magnesium.

Mix the clay with some hydrolat such as rose or lavender water so that it forms a smooth paste, and then paint onto the face. Leave until the mask hardens, then simply wash off with warm water and cotton wool.

While you are waiting for the face mask to set you can set up a crystal grid around the couch or area where the client will be lying.

Cleanse and tone

Cleanse the face using a lotion or cream, and then use a skin toner—rose water or hot water—to wipe off the cleanser. Don't forget you can also add some gem essences to these products if you wish. Once you have

INTERESTING INFORMATION

Origins and History of the Emotional Freedom Technique

EFT was developed by Gary Craig in the early 1990s, although it continues to be refined by many people. It is one of the many forms of meridian energy techniques (METs) now available, and perhaps one of the easiest to learn.

In 1979 acupuncturist Roger Callahan—who had studied applied kinesiology and was an extremely experienced clinical psychologist specializing in phobias, fears and anxieties—was working with a client who had a long-standing phobia of water. Callahan had been studying the subtle energy systems, including meridians, and having already used all the standard psychology tools as well as hypnosis to no avail, he was inspired to ask the client to tap on some meridian points under the eye. His client immediately felt her fear and anxiety disappear. And although many years have now passed, she has remained free of her phobia.

Callahan named this therapy thought-field therapy (TFT).

EFT originated from TFT, and was devised and developed by Callahan in the 1980s. While Callahan developed the basic concept and structure, Craig, who was a student of Callahan, had the vision to refine it and make it accessible to everyone. He also, along with many other therapists working in this field, began to realize the broader possibilities for EFT. As a therapeutic technique there is little else to equal its simplicity and effectiveness. Many experienced therapists now report typical success rates of 80–95% for many conditions. The history of EFT is short; its future looks to be much longer.

Craig refined the technique by simplifying it and using only thirteen main points, which allowed for the possibility of clearing all presenting problems but without the need to have detailed understanding of the meridian system. This meant that the technique could be learned quickly and simply by everyone.

---

ensured that there is no residue of cleanser and that the face is clean you can start the massage.

Crystal face massage

The treatment should be carried out with your client lying on a couch. Ensure that

the client is comfortable and relaxed—if required, have cushions to support his or her back or knees. If the client is cold, you can cover him or her with a blanket. The face should be free of makeup and jewelry. The shoulders should be bare so that you can massage around the neck and shoulder area.

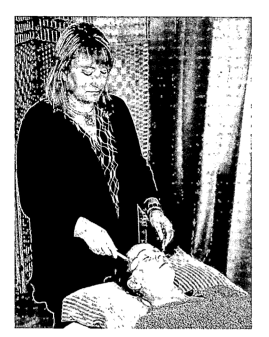

Crystal face massage

Whatever massage oil or other medium you use, ensure that the client's face is well lubricated with the product so that you can glide your fingers/massage tool over the face without dragging the skin.

The illustration shows the step-by-step movements for the Ayurvedic massage. The start point for each movement is indicated by the dots. You gently stimulate these points in a clockwise motion two or three times before following the line with firm pressure, either using your fingers or a massage stone. Generally, when I do this treatment, I start by doing the same movement three times with my fingers and complete the whole procedure. I then use the face mask. During this part of the treatment I will set up the crystal grid I have chosen around the client, and after this I will cleanse the mask and repeat the crystal facial massage, but this time using a crystal rather than my fingers.

During the treatment you can create a rose quartz bath—see the directions for the grid in appendix 2 at the end of the book—and at the end of the treatment you can place some grounding crystals around the couch, as shown in the illustration.

I include a shoulder, arm, and hand massage usually if I have time, but this is optional. I do a final cleanse and then change the crystals to a grounding set.

Grounding layout

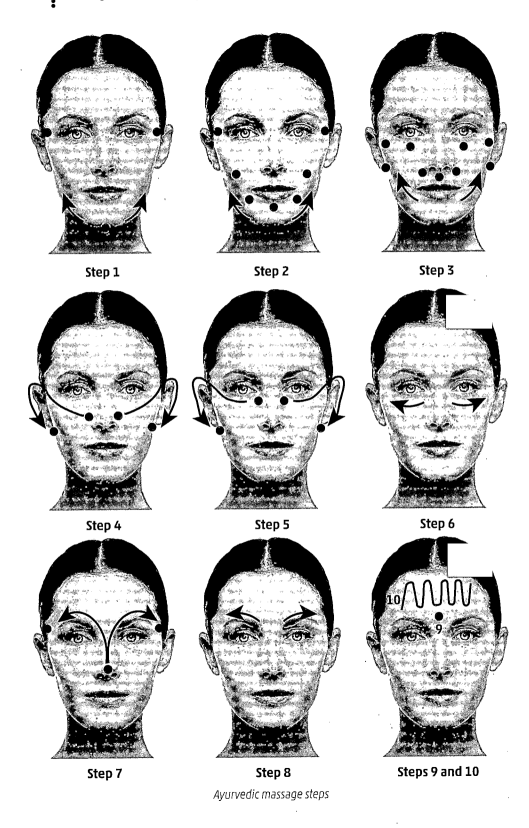

Ayurvedic massage steps

QUESTIONS ON CHAPTER 14

1. Name three contraindications for a facial massage.
2. List the materials you need to carry out a crystal facial.
3. Give three benefits of having a facial.
4. Name the ingredients you would require to prepare a face mask.

CHAPTER 15

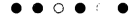

CRYSTALS AND SACRED GEOMETRY

We have already touched upon sacred geometry in chapter 4, where we explored the use of mandalas and the sacred geometry hidden within some of them.

However, there is far more to sacred geometry than mandalas. Many ancient civilizations attached sacred and symbolic correspondences to certain geometric shapes, the mystery schools kept this knowledge secret, and even today "clandestine" societies such as the Freemasons, the Church, and other religious orders use sacred geometry to express their connection with the universe, or God. Scientifically, sacred geometry is illustrated in nature in the way that cells divide and in the way nature recreates patterns— both within our world and beyond all natural growth patterns conform to geometric shapes.

Great works of art have been created by using the golden mean, or golden ratio, to ensure that they have focus and drama. The golden mean is where a line is divided such that the ratio of the whole line to the greater part is the same as the ratio of the greater part to the smaller part. This proportion is found to be particularly pleasing to the eye. Leonardo da Vinci's famous *Mona Lisa* was painted in accordance with the golden mean. Viewers of the painting naturally have

their eyes drawn to the focus of the painting, which is Mona Lisa's face.

Ancient civilizations such as the Mayans, Egyptians, and Greeks constructed buildings using the power of sacred geometry, incorporating it within the architecture of holy buildings such as temples.

In the twelfth century, an Italian mathematician called Leonardo Fibonacci discovered a mathematical sequence that replicated the leaf arrangements in plants, petals in flowers, and patterns in pine cones and shells. In the sequence, the next number is found by adding the two numbers before it: 0, 1, 1, 2, 3, 5, 8, 13, 21, 34, 55, 89, and so on. This system of numbers, Fibonacci discovered, appears everywhere within nature, from the number of flower petals to the pattern of a beehive or scales of a pineapple.

In terms of crystal therapy, however, we are generally more concerned with the energies that are represented within certain geometric shapes and forms.

Crystal therapists use crystals that are carved or faceted into different shapes; there is geometry at work within the seven crystal systems, and when we place crystals around

INTERESTING INFORMATION

- The Greek philosopher and mathematician Pythagoras (*c.* 580–*c.* 500 BC) is the father of sacred geometry. He defined this geometry in expressions of ratios rather than units of numbers.
- The "music of the spheres" is an ancient Pythagorean philosophical concept that the proportions of the sun, moon, and planets create a mathematical pattern that reflects celestial sounds. There are many composers who have explored this concept—Mike Oldfield, Rued Langgaard, Pete Townsend, for example.
- The Platonic solids (tetrahedron, cube, octahedron, dodecahedron, icosahedron) are the basic shapes of sacred geometry and were named after the Greek philosopher Plato (*c.* 429–*c.* 347 BC), who was a student of Socrates and teacher of Aristotle.
- In the 1980s, Dr. Robert Moon of the University of Chicago developed a theory that the ordering of protons and neutrons in the atomic nucleus, and therefore the structure of the periodic table of elements, is based on the Platonic solids.
- Music and numbers connect to sacred geometry. Practitioners of sacred geometry believe that through geometry we can touch God, in the sense that it reflects—via music, arithmetic, and geometry—the order and harmony of creation.

the body in grids or placements there may be sacred geometry created within the treatment. All of this has significance to the energy released from the crystals, especially if we are working consciously with sacred geometry and with intention.

In this chapter, I want to give a broad outline of the energies that common shapes bring once they are incorporated into a crystal or a placement of crystals in grids. For this purpose, in appendix 2 I have added some layouts that incorporate sacred geometry.

It is important to remember that although the essential qualities contained within a crystal don't change, its presenting shape can amplify these properties. So, for example, a crystal in the shape of a wand or crystal point will bring a directional quality to the crystal's energy.

If it is made with rose quartz there will be soft, gentle energy, but a clear quartz wand will present as a sharper, more focused energy. Likewise, a tumble stone will radiate a more diffuse energy, as shown in the diagrams.

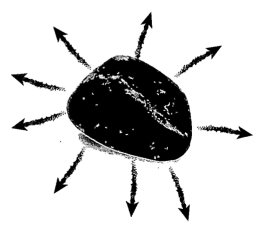

Image of the diffuse outward direction of energy generated by a tumble stone

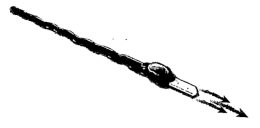

The directional energy flow generated by a crystal point wand

However, it becomes more interesting if we work with other geometric shapes, such as pyramids and spheres. Following is a brief overview of geometric shapes and their correspondences, which you can incorporate into treatments either by creating the shape within your grid or by using crystals of the appropriate geometry.

GEOMETRIC SHAPES AND THEIR CORRESPONDENCES

Pyramid

The pyramid is a sacred shape that is probably best known from those built by the ancient Egyptians, but has also been used by many other ancient civilizations. Its energy is said to be good for amplifying energy and manifestation. It is also an excellent shape to either hold or sit inside when meditating.

Sphere

A balancing energy is generated through spheres; energy is released through a sphere in all directions and therefore is all-encompassing. Meditating with or using a spherical crystal will have a unifying effect.

Obelisks and points

Arguably the most popular shapes of crystals, points and obelisks have an obvious directional flow. If you want to send intentions for manifestation, this shape is perfect for connecting with the universal flow.

Platonic solids

These are named after the ancient Greek philosopher Plato, who explored their meanings in the context of cosmology, theology, and aesthetics. They comprise five shapes, which are reputed to represent cosmic wisdom. It is possible to buy crystal Platonic solid kits. I have found that when used in a grid the treatments generally tend to be more profound. You can use all five or just select the one that you feel is most appropriate for the person receiving the grid.

Attributes of the Platonic solids

Dodecahedron—oneness, unity, unity consciousness, inner peace
Tetrahedron—fire, ambition, masculine, action, focus
Cube, or hexahedron—solidity, strength, order, confinement
Octahedron—inner child, adventure, joy
Icosahedron—new beginnings, feminine, receptive, inner guidance, higher wisdom.

Merkaba

This is sometimes known as a star tetrahedron, or Metatron's cube.

The word comes from three ancient Hebrew words: *Mer*, meaning light; *Ka*, meaning spirit; and *Ba*, meaning body. This shape links us to ascension, the higher self and universal wisdom.

Infinity

The shape of infinity is represented by double-terminated crystals, with attributes of reality beyond the three-dimensional, compassion, and healing.

Spirals

Spirals represent expansion and growth or contraction, depending on directional flow.

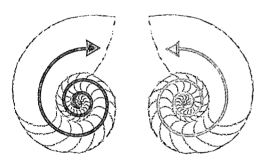

Directional flows of spirals

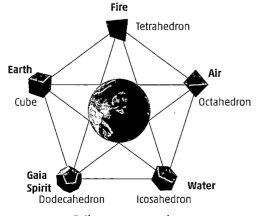

Fire
Tetrahedron
Earth
Air
Cube
Octahedron
Gaia
Spirit
Water
Dodecahedron   Icosahedron

Pythagorean cosmology

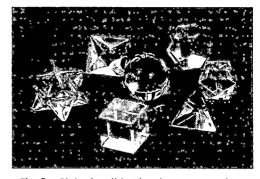

The five Platonic solids. Also shown are a sphere and a merkaba, as these are also included in some Platonic solid crystal sets

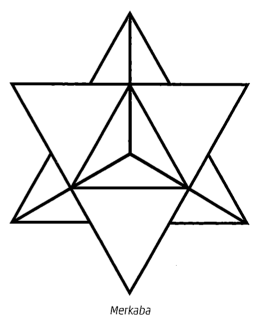

Merkaba

Anyone with an interest in crop circles will be aware of their connection to sacred geometry, and the reiki symbols carry deep symbolic meanings, as do the Om symbol and golden mean. Within this chapter we have only lightly delved into this fascinating subject. I cannot possibly cover it in great depth as that would be a book in itself, but I hope that I have encouraged you to enhance and deepen your ability to work with crystals within the context of sacred geometry.

CRYSTAL TEMPLATES

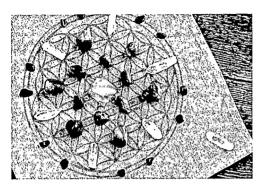

Crystal templates

Another way of using sacred geometry, which seems to be growing ever-more popular, is to use a template of a geometric pattern that you then place crystals upon. The template can be imprinted on cloth, wood, stone, etc., but it is important that the surface is flat. The grid can be placed somewhere to generate a specifically tailored energy, such as during a harvest moon or at a sacred site, you can place it under a couch or chair for healing purposes, or you can simply meditate upon the grid. Obviously, choosing the crystals should be an intuitive process, but you may want to take care to ensure that the crystals you select suit the energy of the pattern you are using.

Templates can be purchased online, or you make them yourself. I have seen cloth templates that have been embroidered and wooden templates that have had an image burned onto them using specialist wood-burning pens (pyrography). If you are using wood, there are specific energy attributes for different types of wood. The colors you use

for the cloth or embroidery will also carry additional energy boosts.

You can also draw or paint your template, or even use mirrors. A simple and cheap method is to download and print a pattern and then glue it onto a piece of paper or board.

There are sacred geometric patterns you can use—here are a few suggestions, along with their correspondences:

Flower of Life

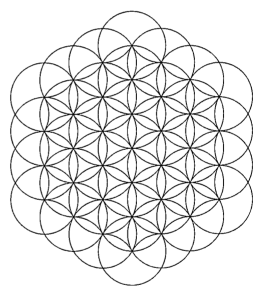

Flower of life

Correspondences: harmony, manifest goals, renewal.

This pattern consists of interweaving circles, which reflects patterns in nature (e.g., flowers, division of cells, etc.).

It is thought to be a good all-purpose pattern that will bring a balancing and manifesting energy to your crystals when they are placed on the grid. Usually they are placed at points of intersection. Within the Flower of Life is a slightly less complex version, the "Seed of Life," which has similar correspondences.

Vesica Pisces

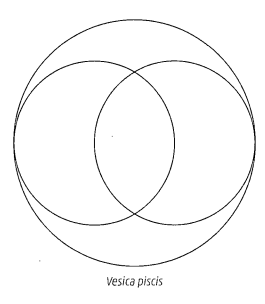

Vesica piscis

Correspondences: connection with and disconnection from others, encouraging understanding.

Seen as the outline of a fish, and commonly used by Christians to represent the coming together of the spiritual and physical worlds. Crystals can be placed intuitively to highlight the shape and intersecting points.

Triangle—sometimes known as Sri Yantra

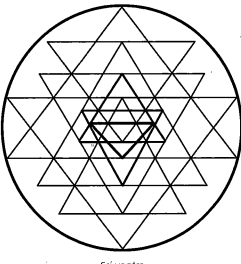

Sri yantra

Correspondences: connection to higher wisdom, grounding new ideas, increasing psychic abilities.

An excellent shape to bring balance and equilibrium.

Square or cube

Correspondences: boundaries, stability, and grounding.

The four corners of the square can be used in sacred geometry to represent the four directions (north, south, east, west), the four elements (earth, wind, fire, water), and the four seasons (spring, summer, autumn, winter).

Circle

Correspondences: friendship, communities, protection.

Traditionally the symbol for unity, which is represented by wedding rings, this shape will also help to promote security and protection.

Star of David

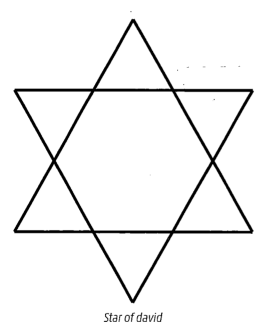

Star of david

Correspondences: uniting spiritual and physical, bringing peace and balance.

Made by two intersecting triangles, the Star of David has its origins in Judaism and is a six-pointed star. This shape is replicated in nature by bees' honeycomb, as well as crystals and frozen water crystals.

REIKI GENERATORS

Reiki generators are a relatively new tool that has appeared and incorporate sacred geometry principles. They have a pyramid sited in the middle of four outward-facing crystal points. I have seen different crystals used, such as rose quartz, clear quartz, and amethyst. They carry the energy of the pyramid, which is upwardly focusing as well as anchoring (representative of bringing energy from spirit to earth), and the clear quartz points are directional, representing perhaps air, fire, earth, and water or north, south, west, and east—this will be determined by the intention of the healer using the grid. The generators are great for enhancing distant healing, and may be placed underneath the couch or chair during a treatment. They can also be placed under specific chakras if you feel they need an extra boost.

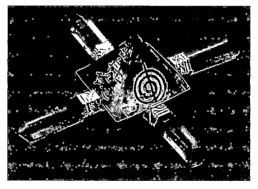

QUESTIONS ON CHAPTER 15

1. Try attuning with different types of crystals that all have the same shape.
2. Can you name the five Platonic solids?
3. What is the music of the spheres?
4. What is this sequence of numbers known as: 0, 1, 1, 2, 3, 5, 8, 13, 21, 34, …?

CHAPTER 16

● ● ○ ● ı ●

CRYSTAL CRAFTS

GROWING YOUR OWN CRYSTALS

This is a lovely exercise to see how crystals form, and is also a good project for children to have a go at.

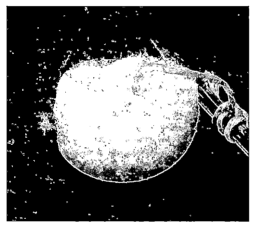

Home-grown crystals

Ingredients

½ cup of tap water
½ cup of salt—Epsom salts or table salt, although table salt takes longer for the crystal to grow and iodized salt doesn't work as well
Small saucepan
String

Pencil
Food coloring (optional)

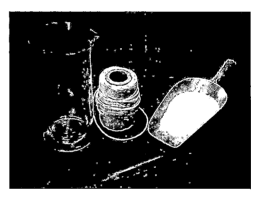

Materials to grow your own crystals

Instructions

Heat the water until it boils, stir in the salt, and remove from heat.
Keep stirring until the water is clear.
Add more salt and keep stirring until you see that the salt grains are no longer dissolving.
Slowly pour the hot water/salt solution into a clean heatproof jar, but don't allow any undissolved grains to fall into the jar.
At this point if you wish you can add food coloring to the mix.

157

Tie the string around the middle of a pencil. You could also add a weight to the string, like a curtain ring or paperclip.

Dangle this in the water about an inch (2.5 cm) or so from the bottom of the jar, and place the pencil along the top of the jar.

Note: crystals will grow only on the string that is in the water, not above the water line.

Leave the jar in a place where it will not be moved or disturbed.

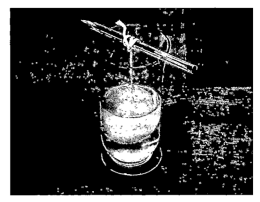

Crystal growing in the jar

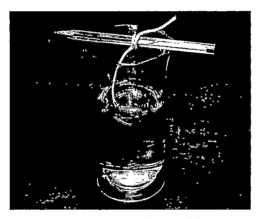

Place the pencil across the top of the jar

If you leave the jar in the sun you will find that the crystals form in a mass. If you place the jar in a cool, shaded place it may grow as a single large crystal. You will also find that if you place a solution made from Epsom salts in the fridge it will grow faster than if you place it in the sun.

Epsom salts will start growing within only a few hours, but table salt may take up to a day or even two before crystals become obvious. However, you should try to leave them for at least two days and up to two weeks to make larger examples.

MAKING A BRACELET

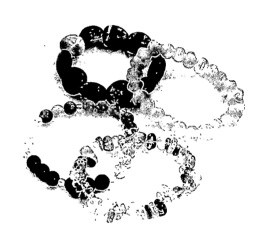

Crystal bracelets

Many people are inspired to use crystals to create personalized bracelets, necklaces, and other jewelry, which look lovely and also generate the healing energies we've discussed in this book.

Here are some ideas and directions to create your own individual pieces of jewelry.

Materials required

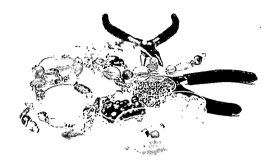

Materials for making a crystal bracelet

Jewelry elastic (this comes in different
    widths—choose one that accommodates
    the size of hole in the beads)
Crystals
Spacer beads
Scissors
Clear nail varnish or jewelry glue

Instructions

1. Cut elastic 1–2 inches (2.5–5 cm) larger
    than the wrist size needed.
2. Select the beads and lay out in the
    pattern that you would like to create.
    Then if you are happy with the design
    you can start to thread the beads onto
    the elastic.
3. Once you have ensured that (a) the
    bracelet is the correct length and (b) that
    the beads are spaced correctly, you are
    ready to finish the piece off.
4. Tie the elastic, ensuring that you can
    place the knot in a bead.
5. Apply clear nail varnish or jewelry glue
    to the knot and allow to dry, then cut off
    the surplus elastic.
6. Move the knot into a bead so it cannot
    be seen.

This is an easy method of making a crystal
bracelet, but the elastic will not last as long
as wire. However, if you make a bracelet
using wire you need to know the exact wrist
size and require a lot more equipment for
fastenings, etc. Note that, depending on the
hardness of the crystals used, they may be
damaged by the wire.

MAKING A CRYSTAL WAND

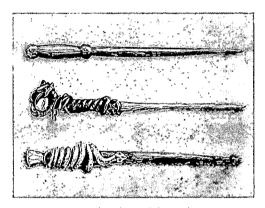

Handmade crystal wands

Materials required

Scissors
Jewelry pliers
Ruler
20 gauge wire of any color you wish
    (although copper is popular as it is
    considered an accelerator of crystal
    energy)
Small branch or stick from a tree of about
    the same thickness as the crystal you
    intend to use for the point of the wand
Quartz crystal about 1.5–2.5 inches
    (4–6.5 cm) long
Beads or smaller crystals for decoration, as
    you choose

Fine-grained sandpaper or unused emery board
Craft knife
Hemp or leather cord

Instructions

1. Select the wood for your wand carefully. Different woods are reputed to have different magically properties:
   a. Oak—divination, healing, manifestation, prosperity, strength, victory
   b. Chestnut—abundance, relieving worry, transforming karma
   c. Yew—death, rebirth, eternity, hallowed ground, shamanic visions.
   It is customary to connect with the tree in much the same way as you would attune to a crystal. Also, some people believe in leaving a small offering to the tree in thanks for what they have taken.
2. Once you have got your stick, strip off the bark with a knife, ensuring that you go along the grain of the wood. Once you have removed the bark, smooth the surface of the wood down by sanding, ensuring that there are no sharp edges. If you want to at this point you can varnish or wax your stick, allowing time for it to dry before completing the next stages.
3. Join the crystal point to the stick by wrapping the wire around them both. The wire should be about 40 inches (100 cm) long. Fold the wire in half around the center of the crystal and twist the two ends together around the stone. Wind or wrap the wire around the stone. Once you get to the bottom of the stone, twist the wire 5 or 10 times. Now continue onto the wood, around 2 inches (5 cm) depending on the size of the wand and crystal.
4. Now reverse, and wrap the wire back upwards from the wood to the crystal.
5. When you get to the crystal, wrap all the ends of the wire as tightly together as you can to help to secure the crystal in place, until you have used up all the wire. You can use the pliers to help tighten the wire around the crystal.
6. To make the handle, cut a roughly 70-inch (175 cm) strip of thin cord or leather. Start to wrap the cord around the bottom of the stick, where you will be holding it. Making sure you wrap the cord tightly around the handle—you can use glue to help secure it. If you wish, you can leave some extra cord and attach beads or feathers to decorate the wand.

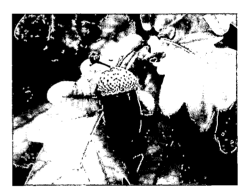

Oak

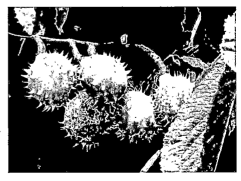

Chestnut

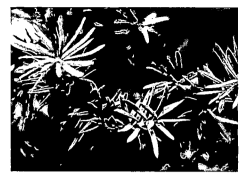

Yew

EXAMPLES OF OTHER CRAFT IDEAS

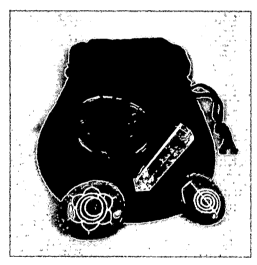

A power pouch

A power pouch is a derivative of the medicine pouches that Native American Indians used. It is usually a small bag—traditionally made of soft leather but you could use any type of soft material or fabric—into which you place a selection of crystals along with other things that relate to the focus that you are creating within the pouch. For example, if you were creating a power pouch for someone who was stressed, you could gather together a selection of crystals that have good stress-busting qualities:

Amethyst for relaxation
Blue quartz for calming
Hematite for grounding
Rose quartz for love

Another idea for a meaningful present is to assemble some crystals together that reflect astrological signs—refer to the birth-stones chart in chapter 9 for ideas of which stones to buy. If you know someone who is going through life changes—like moving, getting married, having a baby, or starting a new job—you could select crystals that reflect the birthstone of the individual, along with crystals that will support the process they are going through. For example, if you know an Aquarian who is having a baby you could select amethyst as the birthstone of Aquarius, a birthstone for the coming baby, some rose quartz for love, and perhaps a gently grounding crystal to anchor the new life on the planet, along with a calming and soothing crystal with angelic energies, such as angelite. You could add a little note with a saying—for example:

When we long for life without difficulties, remind us that oaks grow strong in contrary winds and diamonds are made under pressure.
—**Peter Marshall**

You could also add something from nature, such as acorns or feathers.

RECOMMENDED READING

H. P. Blavatsky, Helena Blavatsy and Michael
Gomes. *Isis Unveiled: Secret of the
Ancient Wisdom Tradition – Madame
Blavatsky's First Work*. Abridged edition.
Quest Books (1997).

Barbara Ann Brennan. *Hands of Light:
Guide to Healing through the Human
Energy Field*. Reissue edition. Bantam
Books (1990).

Donna Eden and David Feinstein. *Energy
Medicine: Balancing Your Body's Energy
for Optimal Health, Joy and Vitality*.
Digital original edition. Piatkus Books
(2008).

C. W. Leadbetter. *Inner Life*. Facsimile of
1910 edition. Society of Metaphysicians
(1999).

Lynne Mctaggart. *The Field: The Quest for
the Secret Force of the Universe*. New
edition. Element (2003).

● ● ◑ ● ◯ ●

CRYSTAL GLOSSARY

AMBER

Amber

Amber is not technically a crystal as it doesn't have a regular atomic structure and therefore has no crystal system; it is classed as amorphous. Nonetheless, many crystal therapists use amber to help balance emotions and also to align us to go with the flow and follow our natural path with positivity.

AMETHYST

Amethyst

One of the most popular stones for beginners and seasoned crystal therapists alike, amethyst helps us to stimulate the upper chakras and connect more deeply with spirit in meditation and treatments. It has protective and healing qualities so is a very good all-rounder. If you only have a few crystals, amethyst is one of the must-haves.

AVENTURINE

Aventurine

Linked to the heart chakra and conditions relating to it, aventurine's calming and soothing green color is good to relieve anxiety and aid personal development and growth. The Church ascribes gems to specific saints, and aventurine is linked with Saint Andrew.

CARNELIAN

Carnelian

A crystal that has a gently nurturing, protective quality, carnelian is also uplifting and can support one during a crisis. The Romans used carnelian to make seals and signet rings, as hot wax does not stick to it. It is also mentioned in the Bible as being used in the breastplates of high priests.

CITRINE

Citrine

Citrine is renowned for its uplifting and energizing qualities. It is a stone that exudes positive vibrations, and many healers feel that it can aid manifestation and abundance.

HEMATITE

Hematite

Hematite has a grounding quality that encourages peace of mind and relaxation. Ancient Egyptians used to place objects made of hematite in tombs. When it is scratched against a white tile, hematite leaves a red line—this is due to its high iron content. However, it is softer than quartz on the Mohs scale—5.5 or 6—so can be scratched by quartz.

RED JASPER

Red jasper

Uplifting yet grounding, red jasper encourages positive thoughts and actions. It is thought to support restful sleep and provides a protective quality as well. Jasper was thought in the past to help gynecological and digestive problems.

LAPIS LAZULI

Lapis lazuli

This is a powerful crystal that was used in ancient Egypt as a cosmetic and also ground into powder and placed into the brow chakra by a process known as trepanning (by making a hole in the skull). It is an obvious choice of crystal for the brow chakra, stimulating intuitive thought by calming and stilling the mind.

MALACHITE

Malachite

Malachite is a powerful crystal that works especially well on the heart chakra and stimulates release of deep-seated emotions or beliefs. It is considered to be a stone that helps transformation of mind, body, and spirit.

MOONSTONE

Moonstone

This crystal has a feminine quality and can be used to support any conditions associated with the female monthly cycle. It is also used to empower wishes and desires. It gets its name from the Romans, who considered that it was formed from moonlight, and in India it is still prized as a sacred stone.

OBSIDIAN

Obsidian

Aiding clear thinking and insight, obsidian is a glass that is formed when lava from volcanoes cools rapidly. Although it is fragile (5 on the Mohs scale) and easily broken, it was used by many ancient civilizations to create sharp implements, such as arrowheads and knives.

PYRITE

Pyrite

Pyrite is a stone that can aid grounding but also empowers an individual at the same time. It has protective qualities and is a great stone to place on your desk to help focus and stimulate intellect.

BLUE QUARTZ

Blue quartz

This crystal is growing in popularity due to the scarcity of blue lace agate, which has been over-mined and is now becoming much harder to source. Many healers use blue quartz as a crystal for the throat chakra.

CLEAR QUARTZ

Clear quartz

Clear quartz is said to contain all the colors of the spectrum, so can be used to balance and realign any chakra. It is also a good choice when you wish to program crystals to emit specific energies. Clear quartz emits an energizing and clarifying energy. It is good for focus and sustaining attention to detail.

ROSE QUARTZ

Rose quartz

The first "go-to" stone for most crystal enthusiasts, this crystal has qualities of unconditional love. It is an excellent crystal to display in a treatment room or bedroom, and can be programmed to attract love and joy.

SMOKY QUARTZ

Smoky quartz

Smoky quartz has an absorbing quality that enables effective grounding and protection of the energy field. It has been used as a gemstone to decorate ornamental and religious objects for thousands of years.

SNOWY QUARTZ

Snowy quartz

Another feminine stone, snowy quartz contains a purifying energy that can help cleanse every chakra or the auric field. It helps us to stay balanced and generates a calm, stable energy.

SODALITE

Sodalite

A crystal often associated with the brow chakra and its correspondences, such as insight, meditation, and intuition. Sodalite can help connection with guides and promote stillness to enable effective communication with spirit.

TIGER'S EYE

Tiger's eye

Tiger's eye has a masculine quality, aiding courage and stamina in the face of conflict and upset. It has a protective quality, and Roman soldiers were said to wear it when they were going into battle.

BLACK TOURMALINE

Black tourmaline

Black tourmaline is sometimes known as schrol. In medieval times, it was used to treat physical and mental disorders. Today, crystal healers use black tourmaline for its strong grounding and protective qualities, as well as using it to dispel fear and negative thoughts. It also comes in pink and green, and a crystal with a combination of both pink and green is known as watermelon tourmaline.

TURQUOISE

Turquoise

A crystal that has been used extensively by ancient civilizations through the ages, from Egypt through to Native American Indians, turquoise is an excellent stabilizer of emotions. It brings serenity, empathy, and wisdom. It is a stone that can be used on the chakra located at the thymus, which links to both the heart chakra and the throat chakra.

● ● ○ ● ◡ ●

CRYSTAL GRIDS

The following is a suggested list of placements of crystals to form crystal grids. These can be used by placing crystals around the body of someone lying on the floor, on a yoga mat, or on a couch. I encourage my students *not* to place crystals on the body, as they work just as well when used within the aura (after all, even the chakras are not directly on the body), and using them this way ensures that recipients of the treatment can drift off into a calm and relaxing meditative state instead of being conscious of the weight of the crystals upon them or being concerned that they may displace the crystals they are "wearing." In addition to this, I have found that recipients are also then more likely to be able to become aware of the energy changes and shifts that are working within their energy system, when the physical presence of the crystal has been taken away.

These grids can also be used as distant-healing layouts, and for this should be placed around a photograph of the person you are sending the healing to.

CRYSTAL COLOR BATHS

● ● ● ● ● ● ● ○ ○ ○ ● ● ● ● ◌ ○ ◔ ● ● ●

This is a good exercise to help you sensitize to the different energies of color. Begin by first cleansing six crystals of the same color under running water. Then place the crystals at the head, shoulders, hips, and feet. Visualize the crystals generating the energy of the color, surrounding and encompassing you with its vibrational frequency, and allow this energy to gently drift into your aura. Try to relax, breathing in through the nose and out through the mouth, and focus on the qualities that you can feel generating from the crystals and their colors. Once you have finished, remove the crystals and cleanse them. Ensure that you are fully grounded afterwards.

This exercise can be repeated with a complementary color—a color that is the opposite to the initial color (see the color wheel in chapter 4). The shadow of a green object will contain some red.

Green color bath grid

This provides a regenerating, peaceful energy bath. Use six green aventurine crystals. You should visualize the energy they generate as vibrant.

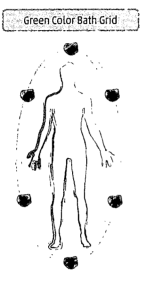

Red color bath grid

This provides a stimulating, activating energy bath. Use six red jasper crystals. Visualize the energy they generate as vibrant and stimulating.

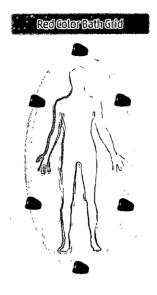

Blue color bath grid

This provides a soothing, serene energy bath. Use six blue quartz crystals. Visualize the energy they generate as calming and soothing.

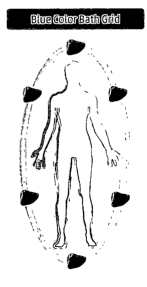

Yellow color bath grid

This provides a stimulating and strengthening energy. Use six yellow tiger's eye crystals. Visualize a soft yellow energy.

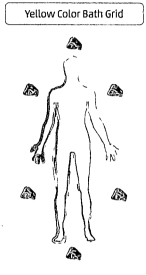

Yellow Color Bath Grid

Purple color bath grid

This provides spirituality and purification, making a calming and restorative energy bath. Use six amethyst crystals. Visualize the energy as deep purple.

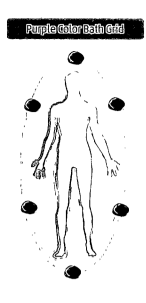

Purple Color Bath Grid

Black color bath grid

This provides an energy bath that has protective, grounding, and absorbing qualities. Use six black tourmaline crystals. Visualize the energy as encouraging protection and grounding of the energy field.

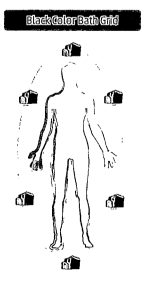

Black Color Bath Grid

Orange color bath grid

This provides an invigorating and vitalizing energy bath. Use six carnelian crystals. Visualize the energy as soft and orange.

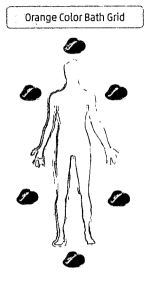

Orange Color Bath Grid

Indigo color bath grid

This provides an energy bath suitable for meditation and creative thought processes, encouraging restful sleep. Use six sodalite crystals. Visualize the energy as deep indigo.

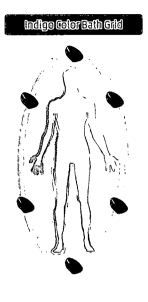

Indigo Color Bath Grid

Rose quartz bath grid

This provides an energy bath of unconditional love. Use six rose quartz crystals. Visualize the energy as soft pink.

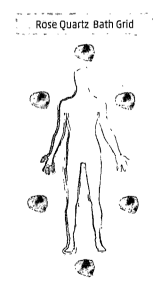

Rose Quartz Bath Grid

REIKI EMPOWERMENT GRID

This grid can be used during a reiki treatment to support the reiki flow and create an ambient atmosphere for deep healing and relaxation.

You will need six amethyst "teeth" and one pyrite cube.

Begin by first cleansing all the crystals— if you are reiki 2 you can use the power symbol. Place the amethyst at the head, shoulders, thighs, and feet, pointing outward, with the pyrite cube placed at the solar plexus. If you wish you can use your reiki to activate the crystals before beginning your reiki treatment.

Try to relax and concentrate on the reiki energy. You should find the flow and quality of energy enhanced. Once you have finished, remove the crystals and cleanse them. Ensure that you and your client are fully grounded afterward.

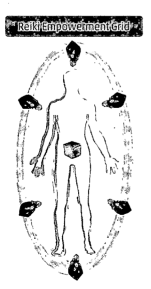

Reiki Empowerment Grid

ENERGY REFRESH GRID

This helps to release stagnated or excess energy from the aura.

You will need six clear quartz single-terminated crystals.

Begin by first cleansing the crystals. Then place the crystals with points **outward** to release stagnant energy. After five to ten minutes, you can reverse the crystals if you wish to simply clear the aura, perhaps before continuing the treatment with a different configuration of crystals. Alternatively, you can turn the crystals so that the points face **inward** to recharge the energy field. Always cleanse the crystals before you start, but also in this case as you change them over. Be aware of how you feel during this process. It is not uncommon to find that the charging process needs less time than the cleansing, but reactions always vary and are individual.

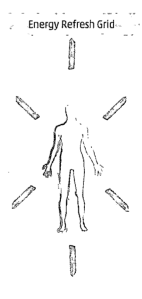

Energy Refresh Grid

PLATONIC SOLIDS GRIDS

Tetrahedron

Element: Fire
Direction: South (if you wish you can place the grid facing south)
State: Heat
Crystals: 3 × carnelian
Keywords: Inner guidance

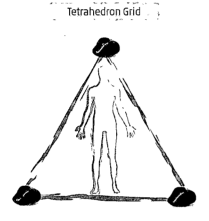

Tetrahedron Grid

Dodecahedron

Element: Universe
Direction: Centre
State: Ether
Crystals: 5 × amethyst
Keywords: Balance, equilibrium, and deep healing

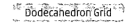

Dodecahedron Grid

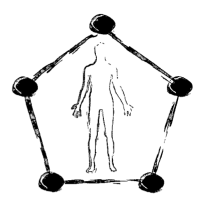

Cube, or hexahedron

Element: Earth
Direction: North (if you wish you can place the grid facing north)
State: Solid
Crystals: 4 × pyrite
Keywords: Centering and grounding

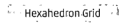

Hexahedron Grid

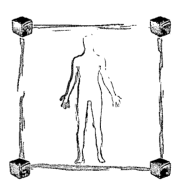

Icosahedron

Element: Water
Direction: West (if you wish you can place the grid facing west)

State: Liquid
Crystals: 6 × blue calcite
Keywords: Transformation and release

Icosahedron Grid

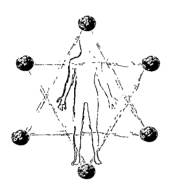

Octahedron

Element: Air
Direction: East (if you wish you can place the grid facing east)
State: Gas
Crystals: 4 × clear quartz
Keywords: Protection and transmutation

Octahedron Grid

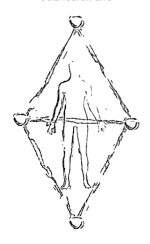

ANGELIC EMPOWERMENT GRID

Use this crystal placement to help you connect with the angelic realms. Angels draw closer in times of need and offer support, love, and protection.

You will need five snowy quartz crystals and one clear quartz crystal.

Begin by first cleansing all the crystals. You can do this by visualizing white light passing through the crystals if you wish.

Place the white snowy quartz crystals around the body at intervals as shown in the picture. Then place the clear quartz crystal either by the crown or under the couch in line with the solar plexus area of the client. Visualize or ask that the crystals become activated and then "hold" the energy with your hands. You should become aware of the energy field changing as the frequencies from the crystals come into play. You can activate the crystals for yourself and step into the grid in order to meditate or receive angelic healing.

Angelic Empowerment Grid

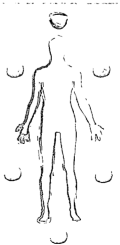

ELECTROMAGNETIC GRID

This grid uses shungite, which is a powerful mineral from Russia renowned for its protective qualities in relation to electromagnetic frequencies.

You will need three shungite crystals and three white agate crystals.

Begin by first cleansing all the crystals. You can do this by visualizing white light passing through the crystals if you wish.

Place the white agate crystals around the body at intervals, as shown in the picture. Then place the shungite in between each piece of white agate. Visualize or ask that the crystals become activated and then "hold" the energy with your hands. You should become aware of the energy field changing as the frequencies from the crystals come into play. You can activate the crystals for yourself and step into the grid in order to meditate or receive healing.

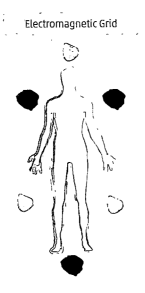

Electromagnetic Grid

LOW ENERGY GRID

Use this grid when you are feeling "out of sorts," tired, or demotivated. Citrine has an enlivening quality that also helps to make you feel uplifted and positive.

You will need four quartz crystal points and four citrine crystals.

Begin by first cleansing all the crystals. You can do this by visualizing white light passing through the crystals if you wish.

Place the citrine crystals around the body at intervals as shown in the picture. Then place the quartz points in between, with the pointed end of the crystal pointing inward (if you wish you can start this grid by positioning the quartz points outward so that you draw off stagnant energy and then reverse the points inward to recharge). Visualize or ask that the crystals become activated and then "hold" the energy with your hands. You should become aware of the energy field changing as the frequencies from the crystals come into play. You can activate the crystals for yourself and step into the grid in order to meditate or receive healing.

Low Energy Grid

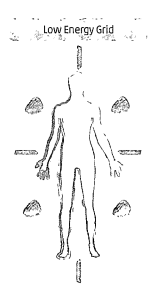

could then replace the red jasper with rose quartz and reverse the quartz points to replace the energy that has been drawn off with a more positive, comforting energy). Visualize or ask that the crystals become activated and then "hold" the energy with your hands. You should become aware of the energy field changing as the frequencies from the crystals come into play. You can activate the crystals for yourself and step into the grid in order to meditate or receive healing.

Release Anger Grid

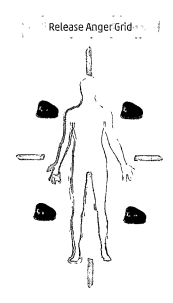

RELEASE ANGER GRID

Use this grid when there are unresolved anger issues at play. It is always good to see if you can determine where the anger is being held in the body—common points that can hold energy are the throat chakra (unexpressed anger), solar plexus chakra (personal power issues), heart chakra (low self-esteem or lack of love), and brow chakra (recurring thoughts and emotions).

You will need four clear quartz crystal points and four red jasper crystals.

Begin by first cleansing all the crystals. You can do this by visualizing white light passing through the crystals if you wish.

Place the red jasper crystals around the body at intervals, as shown in the picture. Then Place the quartz points in between, with the pointed ends of the crystals pointing outward (if you wish, after allowing the crystals time to connect and discharge the energies, you

GRID LAYOUTS FOR THE SUBTLE BODIES

Technique 1

Choose seven crystals intuitively—one for each subtle body—and place them at the side of the recipient, who can lie or sit. Place the crystal relating to the etheric body nearest to the physical body and then work away from the body, placing each crystal where you feel it is the most appropriate for the subtle body it is working on. This technique "separates" the subtle bodies and makes it easier for the healer to feel where one body starts and another finishes. As you go through the layers you may feel differences in temperature, pressure, and quality between each subtle body. It also allows the healer to focus on one body that requires healing.

Technique 2

This is good for self-healing. Place the seven crystals as before but focus on each one in turn and use the breath to breathe energy from the relevant crystal into the aura. If it helps, you can visualize the energy as a colored mist or shield of light. However, do be very clear that this is working on the subtle bodies and not the chakras.

Technique 3

Use appropriate crystal "baths" for each subtle body. Some examples of crystals you could use are:
Etheric body—6 × carnelian
Emotional body—12 × smoky quartz
Mental body: 3 × clear quartz and 3 × sodalite or lapis—it may also help to lay a lapis or sodalite on the brow chakra
Spiritual body—3 × kunzite or danburite and 3 × amethyst.

Grids for the subtle bodies

The etheric

For anyone wishing to see energy, the etheric body is the easiest to perceive. It

is often described as looking like a heat haze around the body, or occasionally lit up as though there were a lamp around the person's head. This is believed to be the origin of the halos that appear around the heads of saints and angels. This energy field is affected by shock, drug use, and any unresolved energy blockages that filter down from the other subtle bodies. It is the nearest subtle body to the actual physical body, is connected to the base chakra, and contains a blueprint of the physical body.

Keywords for when this body is out of balance: Lack of energy, feeling ungrounded, weak and exhausted.

Crystals for this grid: 5 × citrine and 5 × red jasper tumble stones.

Place crystals alternately interspersed in the auric field approximately 0–2 inches (0–5 cm) away from the physical body.

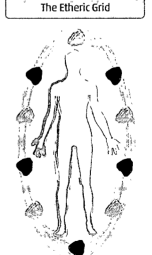

The Etheric Grid

The astral body, or emotional body

Contained between the etheric body, this subtle body holds emotions and memories from both this lifetime and others that are specific to the individual. This subtle body is aligned to the fourth dimension and beyond, and can hold the memory of past-life trauma, which in turn can create surprisingly strong emotional reactions to events that occur in this lifetime that resonate with that trauma. As it is linked to the sacral chakra it empowers thought and intention as well as emotional stability.

Keywords for when this body is out of balance: Emotional overreaction.

Crystals for this grid: 5 × carnelian and 5 × blue sodalite tumble stones.

Place crystals alternately interspersed in the auric field approximately 1–3 inches (2.5–7.5 cm) away from the physical body.

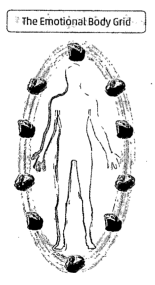

The Emotional Body Grid

The lower mental body

Following on from the emotional body, the lower mental body receives, holds, and conveys thoughts, beliefs, and mental processes, which link very much to the reality we create. Our conscious and unconscious beliefs impact on the life we experience. When it is functioning well this subtle body creates rational and clear thinking. It is linked to the solar plexus chakra.

Keywords for when this body is out of balance: Overactive mind, insomnia, and brain fog.

Crystals for this grid: 5 × tiger's eye and 5 × clear quartz tumble stones.

Place crystals alternately interspersed in the auric field approximately 3–8 inches (7.5–20 cm) away from the physical body.

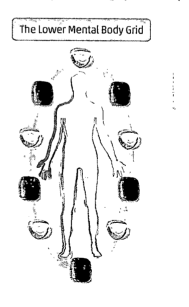

The Lower Mental Body Grid

The higher mental body, or astral body

This subtle body acts as the bridge between the spiritual and physical realm and holds the aspects of the personality. It is within this body that we gain inspiration and healing energies from spirit, which are then disseminated into the other subtle bodies. The higher mental body is linked to the heart chakra.

Keywords for when this body is out of balance: Inability to be at peace with oneself or others.

Crystals for this grid: 5 × rose quartz and 5 × green aventurine.

Place crystals alternately interspersed in the auric field approximately 6–12 inches (15–30 cm) away from the physical body.

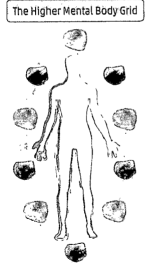

The intuitional body, or causal body

The causal body is what links us to the collective consciousness. It contains the gifts and talents that we have gained in previous lives that are waiting to be unlocked in this life when the soul decides the time is right. This subtle body is linked to the throat chakra but also to the causal chakra, which is sited at the back of the head and is one of the new transpersonal chakras.

Keywords for when this body is out of balance: Fear of death, insecurity, paranoia.

Crystals for this grid: 5 × aquamarine and 5 × apophyllite.

Place crystals alternately interspersed in the auric field approximately 12–24 inches (30–60 cm) away from the physical body.

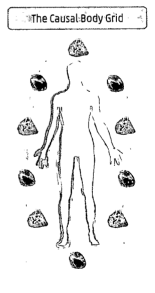

The spiritual body, soul body, or celestial body

Contained within this subtle body is the very essence of your spirit and your connection to your soul or higher self, or, as some would say, the God essence, which everyone who incarnates physically brings with them. It filters spiritual inspiration and understanding into the lower chakras. The soul body is linked to the brow chakra.

Keywords for when this body is out of balance: Disconnection from soul and universe.

Crystals for this grid: 5 × clear quartz and 5 × blue sodalite.

Place crystals alternately interspersed in the auric field approximately 24–30 inches (60–75 cm) away from the physical body.

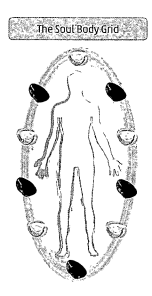

The Soul Body Grid

The divine body, integrated spiritual body, or ketheric template

This is the subtle body where all the others converge, and it integrates the energies. Although it is the subtle body that is furthest away from the physical body, it contains an energy line that flows up and down the spine, linking all the chakras and circulating energy throughout the whole system. This subtle body is linked to the crown chakra.

Keywords for when this body is out of balance: Separation of physical and spiritual existence.

Crystals for this grid: 5 × apophyllite and 5 × amethyst tumble stones. If you have one, this placement will be further enhanced by a merkaba-shaped crystal.

Place crystals alternately interspersed in the auric field approximately 30–44 inches (75–110 cm) away from the physical body.

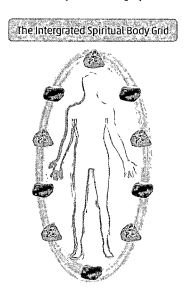

The Intergrated Spiritual Body Grid

APPENDIX 3

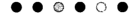

CRYSTAL ATTUNEMENT SHEETS

CRYSTAL ATTUNEMENT SHEET

Your interpretation of the significance and uses of this crystal – *give at least three:*

Crystal Name:	Family Group Name:

Crystal System:	Chemical Composition:

Countries of Origin:	Hardness:

Crystal Formation:

Colors:

Other Significant Information – Special care, poisonous, contra-indications:

Meanings – from at least three different sources: please continue overleaf

---

APPENDIX 4

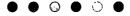

THE MANDALA

MANDALA DIAGRAM

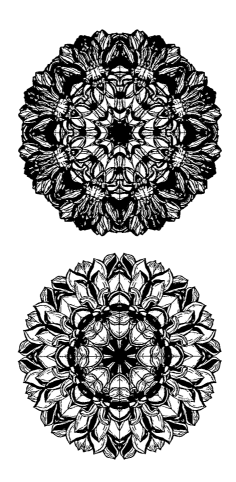

INTERPRETING THE MANDALA

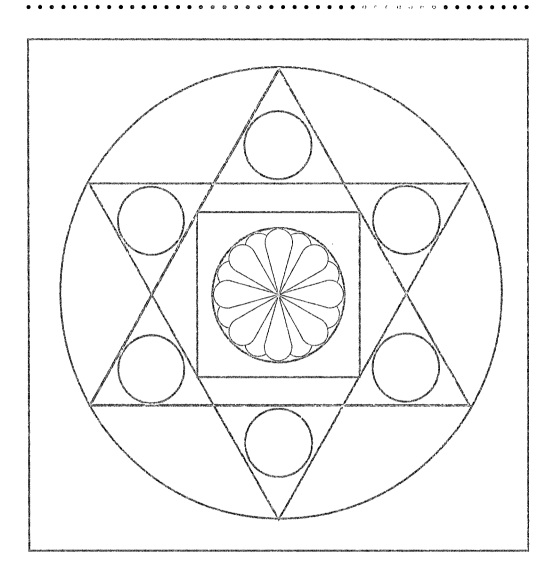

Some people find that they can interpret the mandalas of others. Looking at it in the following way you may be able to feed back to the person who has drawn it.

If the square has been colored in, it could indicate that the person who created the mandala is grounded. To what extent they are grounded might be indicated by the color they used in the square.

The "star" shape indicates the part of the person that is projected to others. If the "arrows" of the star and the spheres inside the arrows are colored in an ordered way, this might suggest someone who is in control, ordered, calm, etc. Or it might indicate that the person is very conventional and doesn't like to try new things or take risks. If it is colored in a disordered way with lots of different colors, it could indicate someone who is perhaps at best creative with a lot going on, or alternatively someone who is quite chaotic and busy. Again, the colors might give an indication as to where the balance lies.

The "flower" in the center can indicate the "hidden" self—it could indicate the spiritual aspect of the person, the subconscious, or just the aspects of the person that wouldn't normally be shown to other people. There is the potential for "boundaries" to be drawn in around the "flower," which might indicate a person in need of protection, someone who is very good at keeping this center hidden from others, or someone who likes to keep people at arm's length.

When doing this exercise, just let your mind go into a calm, meditative state and see what you feel comes up.

The mandala can be used as Jung used it, for personal insight, but you can also use it as a healing tool by placing crystals where you feel the energies need to be highlighted and using it as a grid layout.

Again, choose your crystals for the mandala grid instinctively and have your partner hold the energy of the grid for at least ten minutes or longer.

Red is the color of blood and of life. It is the color of pain and passion, which come with the initiation of change.

Yellow is precise and optimistic, for clear and incisive decisions. The whirling, intellectual, rational side of our being.

Blue represents a place of stillness and strength, tranquility, and calm from which we express our dreams and our purpose.

Orange represents choosing the right beginnings and the determination to move forward into the light and away from the dark. It also encourages childlike joy of living in the moment without doubt or fear.

Green is for growth, harmony, and stability. This generous color is the color of innocence and joy, where something new is beginning to form.

Purple is an aristocratic color representing transformation of the past, and the faith and knowledge in our own inner center.

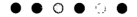

CRYSTAL CASTING BOARDS

Select crystals of your choice, which hold significant meaning for you, or you could use a rainbow chakra set. Here are a few suggestions of keywords for some crystals you may wish to use:

Amethyst—spiritual growth/transformation
Aventurine—emotional issues/change
Citrine—upliftment and abundance
Clear quartz—clarity/purpose
Rose quartz—love/harmony
Red jasper—grounding/manifestation
Snowflake obsidian—protection/support
Blue quartz—communication/insight

Add any other crystals that contain meaning for you to the mix that you use—store them in a pouch and use them only for the purpose of using the board. Remember to cleanse before and after use.

Directions for use:

1. Ground and center yourself.
2. Think of the questions/issues you would like to focus on.
3. "Cast" the crystals—some people simply rub the crystals together between both hands, or just hold them to tune into the crystals and ask for guidance.
4. Holding your hand above the chart, drop the crystals onto the chart—try not to hold your hand over any specific areas of the chart as they fall.
5. Discard the crystals that fall outside of the chart.
6. Now look closely at which sections the crystals have fallen into.
7. Try to "read" the correlation between the area of the chart the crystal has fallen onto and the correspondence for the crystal—if you have mastered the ability to attune to a crystal with confidence you will find that the information flows in much the same way as reading a tarot card.

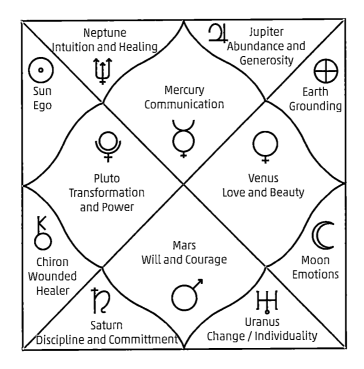

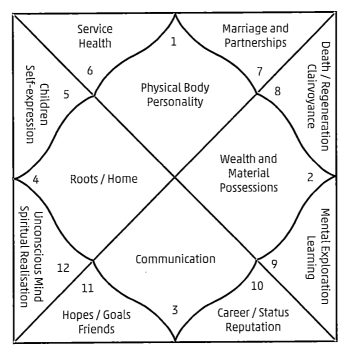

Crystal casting boards

● ● ○ ● ◌ ●

DOWSING CHARTS

The following charts are to help you assess answers to questions requiring numbers, such as "How many drops of essence should I take?" *yes/no* answers, and so on. It is important first of all to see if you can get your pendulum to show you a *yes/no* answer, which for most people is demonstrated by it swinging in a particular direction for *yes* and another direction for *no*. In my case, my pendulum swings clockwise for *yes* and anticlockwise for *no*, but it also swings backwards and forwards to indicate a neutral or "not appropriate to answer" response. When you are using charts, most people find the best way is to hold the pendulum over the chart and to wait for it to start to swing towards a particular answer. So when using pendulums with charts, instead of giving a *yes/no* answer the pendulum will swing in the direction of the correct answer on the chart.

For some people the pendulum will respond very quickly when they first start to dowse, but for others it can be a frustrating process. I have found that people with analytical, questioning mindsets find it harder to start to dowse than those whose disposition is more likely to allow them to "go with the flow" or just see what happens. With patience everyone can dowse. If you are struggling with dowsing do not try to do it when you are under pressure to make it work. Put the pendulum aside and try again another time. It is good to try to make sure that you are balanced, and a short meditation to align each chakra by visualizing different colors relating to the chakras or by holding some chakra crystals and just sitting with them for a few minutes will help to do this. When you ask questions, try to forget about what possible answers there could be and allow the pendulum to try to work independently of your mind!

No one really understands how dowsing works—they just know that it does! For many years it has been used by people, for example, to locate water, and it is a method trusted by many. The American Society of Dowsers and the British Society of Dowsers both aim to further the knowledge and understanding of dowsing, so for people who are interested in dowsing, their websites are a good resource—www.dowsers.org and www.britishdowsers.org.

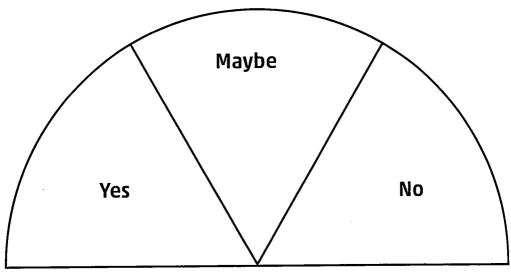

Dowsing chart

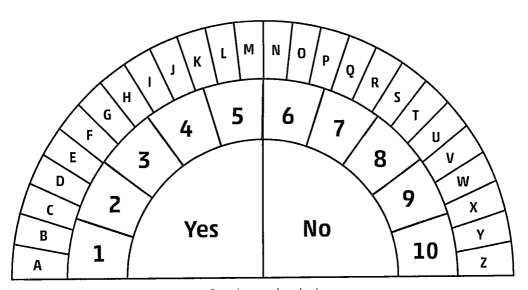

Dowsing number chart

INDEX